THE WHEAT- & DAIRY-FREE COOKBOOK

THE WHEAT- & DAIRY-FREE COOKBOOK

TERENCE STAMP   ELIZABETH BUXTON

PHOTOGRAPHY BY JONATHAN LOVEKIN

EBURY
PRESS
LONDON

First published in 1997 as The Stamp Collection Cookbook
Paperback edition published in 2000

This new edition published in 2002

  3 5 7 9 10 8 6 4 2

First published in 1997 by Ebury Press, Random House,
20 Vauxhall Bridge Road, London SW1V 2SA

Random House Australia (Pty) Limited, 20 Alfred Street, Milsons Point,
Sydney, New South Wales 2061, Australia

Random House New Zealand Limited, 18 Poland Road, Glenfield,
Auckland 10, New Zealand

Random House South Africa (Pty) Limited, Endulini, 5A Jubilee Road,
Parktown 2193, South Africa

Random House Group Limited Reg. No. 954009
www.randomhouse.co.uk

A catalogue record for this book is available from the British Library

ISBN 0 09 188893 X

Editing: Susan Fleming and Anne McDowall
Design: Michael Nash Associates
Photography: Jonathan Lovekin
Food stylist: Catharine Calland
Stylist: Nato Welton
Authors' photograph: Terry O'Neill

Printed and bound in Portugal by
Printer Portuguesa L.d.a.

TABLE OF CONTENTS

INTRODUCTION BY
TERENCE STAMP
7

INTRODUCTION BY
ELIZABETH BUXTON
9

SOUPS, STARTERS,
VEGETABLES AND
SALADS   11

VEGETARIAN MAIN
DISHES
49

FISH
73

FOWL
93

COOKIES, CAKES
AND DESSERTS
117

BASICS
145

ACKNOWLEDGMENTS
156

FLOUR
157

INDEX
158

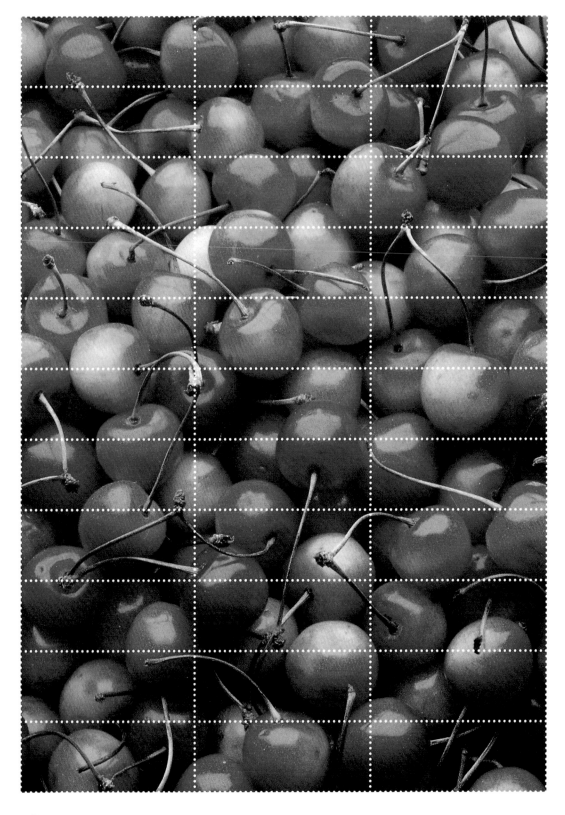

INTRODUCTION BY TERENCE STAMP

Foodies, be warned. You are about to enter a sugar-free, wheat-free, dairy-free and salt-free zone. This is not a cookbook for fainthearts or faddists. Such people will find little to solace them in these pages. But for those who have the capacity for experiment, and the gumption to persist, I can promise that an abundance of rich rewards and tasty treats lies just ahead.

When, in 1994, Elizabeth Buxton and I launched The Stamp Collection, neither of us, even in optimistic mode, could have predicted the heartening response we received. Suddenly we found ourselves connected to many thousands of people who, through choice or necessity, had turned their backs on some of the common foodstuffs hitherto held to be indispensable. Our numbers in the world, we discovered, were considerable, and growing with every mouthful.

I met Elizabeth Buxton in London when I heard tell of a young girl – Liz's daughter Poppy, who was only nine years old at the time – who could bake marvellous cakes for lost souls like me, forced to address and sustain life without recourse to wheat, dairy and sugar. (I do, by the way, love women who encourage their kids to cook.)

One evening I was invited to dinner chez Buxton, and so our valued friendship began. Not long after that, we observed that Poppy's little sister Lucy was showing signs of the same dietary intolerances as my own. I urged Elizabeth to be as stringent with Lucy's diet as I was with mine. We reminded ourselves, for instance, that even the innocent words 'Natural Flavouring' on a packet of chips might disguise (because there was no legal obligation to specify) unwanted ingredients, such as whey or rusk, capable of sparking eczema. Action was taken and Lucy was soon returned to perfect health.

As a boy in London I ate what the other boys ate: plenty of margarine on toast, jam on toast, dripping (beef fat, and such) on thick slices of bread that could have been used as doorsteps. My mother, like any Mum down our street, knew just how to apply balm to my childhood hurts and traumas: a nice cuppa tea and another gargantuan, fatty doorstep of daily bread.

I loved it all, of course, but none of it loved me back, and though the years passed pleasantly enough there were increasing indications that Something Wasn't Right. Without my knowing it, my body had been kicking up in various ways for decades when, at the age of twenty-seven and with my screen career in the ascent, I finally came up, and down, with my very own special, personal duodenal ulcer which hurt like hell and really got in the way of my life and work.

The road back to feeling good again began for me in Rome, an appropriately inspiring city, where I was filming with the great director Fellini. On the set I enjoyed the services of an Italian interpreter, a charming woman who also happened to be Fellini's regular astrologer. It was this lady who first suggested that all my aches and pains, my sneezes and diseases, were in fact food-based; it was she who encouraged me to adopt a vegetarian diet, to experiment with foods to discover what was right for me, and what was wrong.

And so I embarked on that long, uneasy road that leads home again. The habits of a lifetime had to be unlearned. Most of my favourite comfort foods were henceforth out of bounds. Dismayed, I doubted my staying power. Staying healthy, rejecting what was harmful to me, became a challenge that I would have to face every day for the rest of my life.

But such were the almost instant rewards of health and spirit that the apparently austere requirements of diet became less and less of a chore. Now, of course, it's a way of life. Second nature.

And fun. Plenty of surprises on the way: foods never encountered or even imagined before; browsing in colourful, sweet-smelling fruit and vegetable markets in exotic places; loitering in health shops all over the world, in quest of unusual, even mysterious, tastes and temptations. I was recently in Hawaii with my friends Alice and Henry, in whose garden grew a beautiful breadfruit tree. One night Henry made a wondrous pudding from its fruit, cooked with rice, sweetened with maple syrup, drowned in coconut milk. Miracle time in Hawaii!

I have twice lived on organic farms, the first time on a stretch of rich Spanish earth on the island of Ibiza which belonged to my much missed friend Frederick van Pallandt (of Nina and Frederick singing fame). Together Fred and I returned several acres of his farm to organic culture, and it was surprising and stirring to see how quickly butterflies and birds came back to that enchanted place.

More recently I have lived in a converted windmill on the eastern shores of Long Island, amid many organic fruit orchards. This is where Marilyn Monroe and Arthur Miller honeymooned, and it is indeed a magical hideaway.

Living alone, I often eat alone. An enjoyable experience, I hasten to add. But I also relish the company of friends, particularly perhaps at mealtimes, when the ancient rituals of communal feasting and conviviality may be rediscovered, and the circle closed.

There is, in fact, something sacred about eating together. I feel that Khalil Gibran's line 'Work is love made visible' is particularly applicable to the preparation of food. Offered with love, accepted with grace, food is at the heart of an alchemy that sustains the body and restores the spirit. In my opinion this may be one of the true meanings of the parable of the loaves and fishes, that famous example of simple food being offered, for the good of all by the great healer of souls.

Read and enjoy. Eat and enjoy.

Terence Stamp
Vancouver, 6th June 1997

INTRODUCTION BY ELIZABETH BUXTON

Terence Stamp knows more about food and the effect it has on our well-being, than anyone else I know. Over the years he has introduced me to a style of cooking that focuses on the choice of ingredients and omits wheat, dairy products, sugar and salt.

This book does not intend to 'preach' that everyone should follow this way of eating. Some of us must do so for health reasons, but for the rest of us, a varied diet is always the best.

My daughter Lucy developed food intolerances at six months old, so it was necessary for me to learn to cook without certain ingredients like dairy products derived from cow's milk and to avoid store-bought foods containing peanuts, additives and colourings. It was our friend Terence Stamp who first pointed out that Lucy had a wheat intolerance as well, and suggested that I cook with alternative flours. He has also encouraged me to use sweeteners other than refined sugar and has given us weird and wonderful things, like date sugar and malt powder, with which to experiment. Terence has changed the way we look at food and in so doing has provided this story with a happy ending – Lucy has no more health problems.

The recipes in this book require only a basic knowledge of cooking. The skill is in finding the freshest ingredients and, where ever possible, using organic produce. Cooks wishing to use their normal wheat flour, dairy products or refined sugar can substitute them easily. Salt and lemon juice are both flavour enhancers: our choice is to use lemon juice but yours may be to use salt. Just alter the ingredients to suit your preference.

We have received hundreds of requests to create a Stamp Collection all-purpose wheat-free flour. This was a project waiting to happen. As a cook who has been preparing wheat-free meals for ten years, I have become familiar with a huge array of different flours, each with their own distinctive characteristics: jumbo oats, kibbled oats, malted oats, porridge oats, oatmeal, barley, light rye, dark rye, malted rye, rice, gram, buckwheat, soya, potato, maize meal, millet and unbleached cornflour. Having a store cupboard stocked like this would be impractical for most cooks, so our blend of organic flours is the one used in this book.*

A word about the selection of recipes. Those featured in the first section 'Soups, Starters, Vegetables and Salads' can be served several at a time to make up a smørgåsbord type meal. The only non-vegetarian recipes we have included are for fish and fowl. We have no bones to pick with meat-eaters and everyone is free to make their own choices. This is ours.

Finally, if you think that you may have food intolerances, please be cautious when using any unfamiliar new ingredients that may be found in this book.

*For more information see page 157.

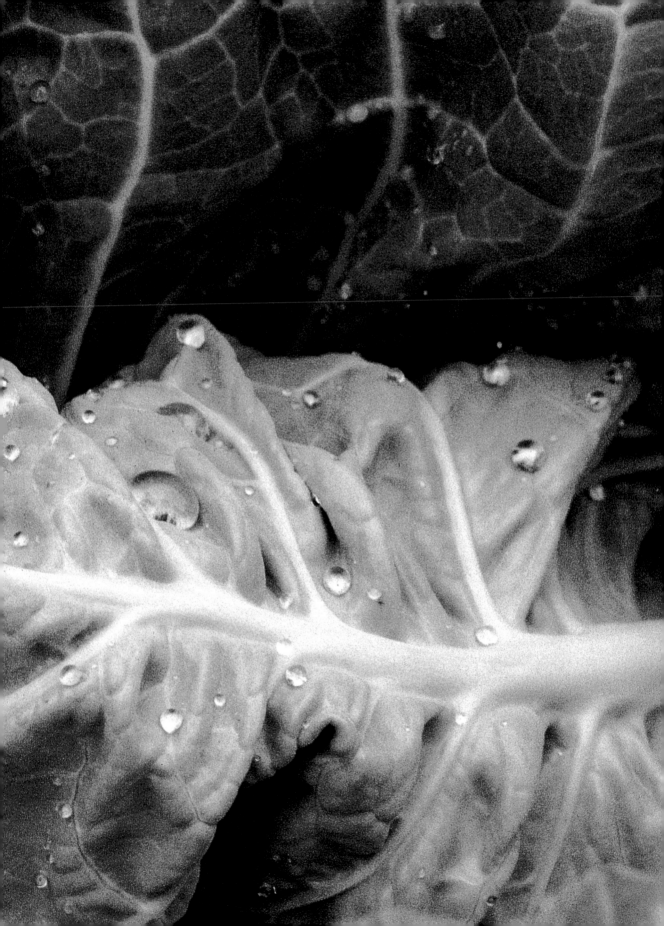

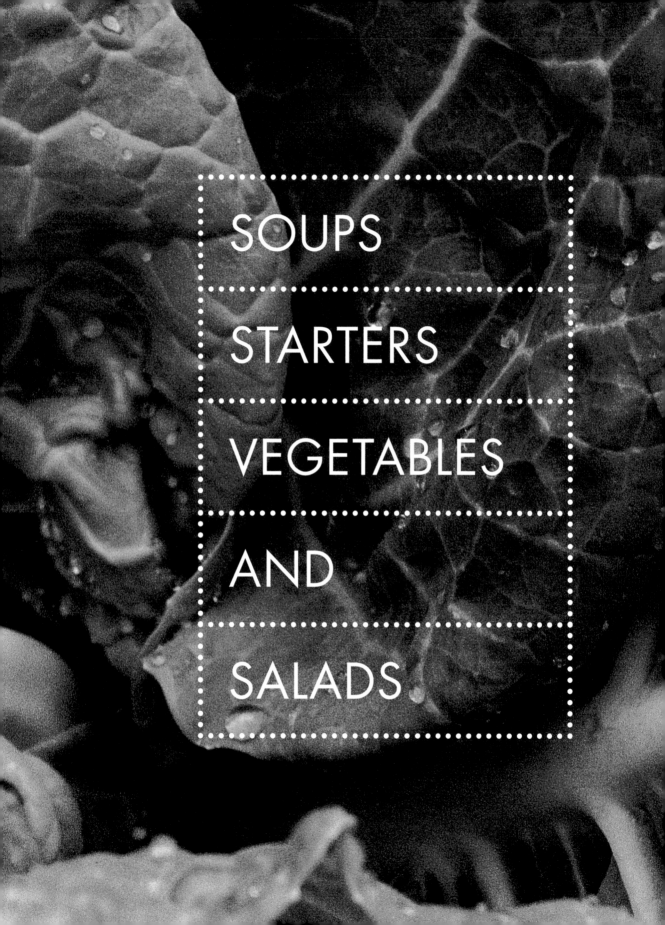

SOUPS

STARTERS

VEGETABLES

AND

SALADS

CLAM CHOWDER

First catch the clams! In the summer time on Shelter Island this is precisely what we do. Lengthy studies of the tide tables followed by hot discussions as to which spot would be the best to visit, picnic planning and alarm clock settings, result in us getting up at dawn, drinks, eats, hats, dry beach towels, sunblock in the beach bag, clamming rakes over the shoulder and buckets in hand. The best clamming spots are those only reachable by boat. This adds to the sense of adventure. We all pile into the dinghy and set off across the water.

Clamming is huge fun for children and adults alike. A certain competition and rivalry arises between the 'teams': one holds the bucket for the clams, the other rakes the sand with the sharply pronged fork. The tines of the fork are spaced quite widely apart so that the small, young clams fall free, and only the larger ones find their way into the bucket. Some of the clams are huge, the size of a fist. These are called quahogs and are traditionally steamed, chopped and used in chowder. The fruits of our clamming expeditions are used for a variety of scrumptious feasts. The smaller clams are eaten raw, the others steamed and used in risottos, sauces, fritters, stuffed in their shells or as this chowder.

	METRIC	IMPERIAL	CUPS
2 quahogs or 20 small clams about 5cm/2in across			
FOR THE BROTH:			
2 whole large cloves garlic			
½ large sweet onion, roughly chopped			
1 large celery stalk, roughly chopped			
1 large carrot, roughly chopped			
2 sprigs fresh thyme			
2 bay leaves			
8 black peppercorns			
olive oil		2 tbsp	
lemon juice		2 tbsp	
water	600 ml	1 pt	2½ cups

	METRIC	IMPERIAL	CUPS
FOR THE CHOWDER:			
olive oil		2 tbsp	
celery, chopped	115 g	4 oz	1 cup
sweet onion, chopped	140 g	5 oz	¾ cup
waxy potatoes, cubed with their skins left on	200 g	7 oz	1 ½ cups
cornflour/cornstarch		3 tbsp	
goat's milk	250 ml	8 fl oz	1 cup
FOR THE GARNISH:			
olive oil		½ tbsp	
chopped celery leaves		2 tbsp	

Put the clams in plenty of cold water and scrub their shells. Change the water from time to time to get rid of the sand. Don't worry about the sand too much because at a later stage in this recipe it will sink to the bottom of the pan of stock where it will remain if the liquid is poured off carefully. Put the vegetables for the broth into a large pan with all the ingredients except for the lemon juice and water. Cook over a gentle heat for 4 minutes without colouring the mixture. Add the lemon juice and water and bring to the boil. Simmer covered for 30 minutes.

Meanwhile prepare the chowder. Put the olive oil, celery and onion into a heavy-based saucepan and cook gently for 5 minutes without colouring, stirring. Add the potato, stir, remove from the heat and then stir in the cornflour and set aside.

Once the broth has cooked for 30 minutes, put in the clams, cover and cook for 5–10 minutes depending upon their size, until the shells open wide. Discard any clams that do not open. Remove the opened clams from the saucepan with tongs, take out the meat and chop roughly. Now strain the broth into the onion, celery and potato mixture. You should have about 600 ml/20 fl oz/2½ cups of broth. Leave the sediment with any sand in the bottom of the broth pan.

Stir the chowder, making sure that the cornflour is incorporated. Add the milk and bring slowly to the boil, stirring. You should now have a smooth mixture that has thickened to the consistency of cream. Add the chopped clams and simmer gently, covered, for 10 minutes or until the potato is just cooked. The vegetables should still be quite firm. Adjust the seasoning to taste. Just before serving, stir in the garnish of olive oil and celery leaves off the heat.

SERVES 4

PEA AND MINT SOUP

Fresh or frozen peas are equally suitable for this recipe. If organic, fresh peas are used, add the emptied pods to the vegetarian stockpot.

	METRIC	IMPERIAL	CUPS
peas (fresh or frozen)	450 g	1 lb	3 cups
1 bunch spring onions/scallions, roughly chopped			
1 head iceberg lettuce, roughly chopped			
good olive oil		2 tbsp	
vegetable or chicken stock (see pages 154 or 155)	900 ml	1½ pints	3¾ cups
1 large sprig mint			
black pepper			
FOR THE GARNISH (optional):			
sheep's yogurt			
mint leaves			

Wilt the peas, onions and lettuce in the olive oil. Add the stock and simmer until the vegetables are tender, about 15 minutes. Liquidize and then add the mint. Add pepper to taste.

For a smoother texture the soup can then be put through a sieve. Garnish with a dollop of yogurt and the mint leaves.

SERVES 4

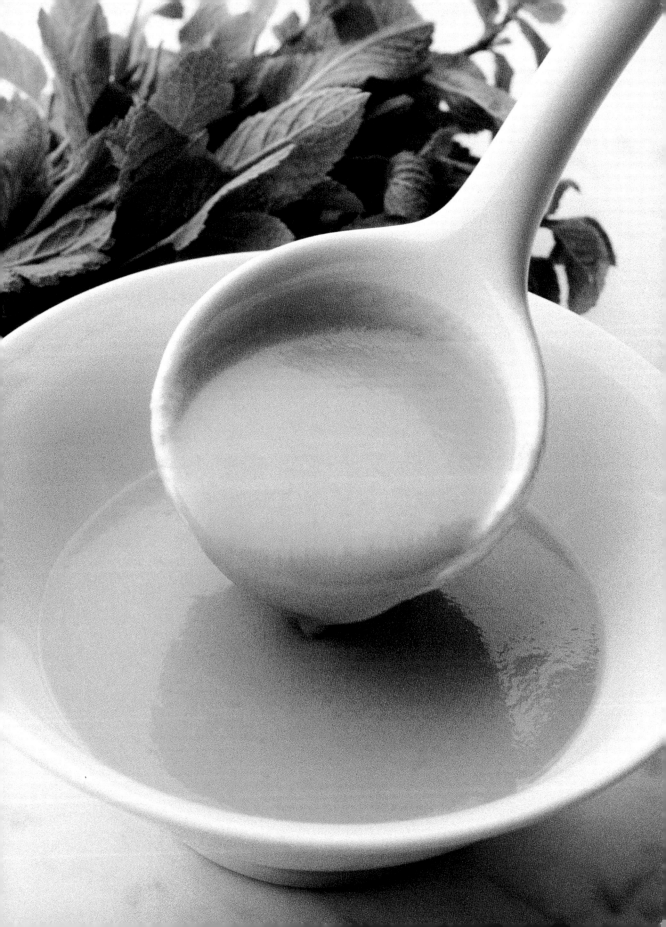

LENTIL SOUP

	METRIC	IMPERIAL	CUPS
lentils	275 g	9½ oz	1⅓ cups
olive oil		2 tbsp	
½ leek, finely chopped			
1 celery stalk, finely chopped			
1 carrot, finely chopped			
1 medium potato, chopped			
lemon juice		1 tbsp	
black pepper to taste			
good vegetarian or chicken stock	1 litre	1½ pt	4 cups
spring onion/scallion tops, to garnish			

Cook the lentils as per instructions on pack.

Heat the oil in a large saucepan. Add the leek, celery and carrot. Cover the pan and cook over a gentle heat for 5 minutes.

Add the potato and cooked lentils, stir, cover and cook for a further 5 minutes. Stir in lemon juice and black pepper. Add stock, bring to the boil, cover and simmer for 30-40 minutes or until vegetables are soft.

Mash lightly with a potato masher to purée some, but not all, of the vegetables. If necessary adjust the seasoning, and add more stock if the soup is too thick.

Serve sprinkled with chopped spring onion tops.

SERVES 4-6

SWEET POTATO AND CARROT SOUP

This is a very clean tasting soup that has a truly amazing colour. Neither orange nor red, it is a brilliant flame colour. Equally delicious hot or cold, this is a useful party standby and makes a refreshing alternative to gazpacho. It may seem from the ingredient list that this is a very spicy soup, but it is not. The blend of flavours is very carefully balanced and no one ingredient dominates.

	METRIC	IMPERIAL	CUPS
olive oil		5 tbsp	
carrots, diced	140 g	5 oz	1 cup
orange-fleshed sweet potato, cut into chunks	140 g	5 oz	1 cup
onion, chopped	115 g	4 oz	2/3 cup
10 green cardamom seeds			
coriander seeds		1 tsp	
3 dried bay leaves			
turmeric or a few saffron strands		1/2 tsp	
lemon juice		1 tbsp	
can chopped tomatoes	1 x 400g	1 x 14 oz	
stock, either vegetable or chicken with any fat removed, (see pages 154 or 155)	500 ml	16 fl oz	2 cups
FOR THE GARNISH:			
sheep's yogurt	100 ml	3 1/2 fl oz	1/2 cup
chopped fresh chives			

In a heavy saucepan heat the oil and cook the carrot, sweet potato and onion for 3 minutes. Add the spices and stir them into the oil for 1 minute. Add the lemon juice, tomatoes and stock, and simmer covered with a lid for 30 minutes, or until the vegetables are tender. Remove the bay leaves and liquidize the contents of the pan in a food processor. Pass the purée through a sieve.

If the soup is to be served hot, pour back into the cleaned saucepan and gently reheat. The soup is meant to be fairly thick, but if you prefer a thinner soup, add a little more stock at this stage. You may then need to adjust the seasoning slightly with a little more lemon juice and black pepper.

If the soup is to be served cold, pour into a bowl, cover and chill in the refrigerator.

Whether hot or cold, garnish with a dollop of the yogurt into which you have whisked the chives.

SERVES 4

SPICY BEAN SOUP

This is my daughter Lucy's recipe. It is a thick soup, robust enough to serve as a light meal. Any beans can be used instead of the ones listed – for example, borlotti, black-eye or chick-peas.

	METRIC	IMPERIAL	CUPS
1 red onion, chopped			
olive oil		4 tbsp	
1 large clove garlic, crushed			
dried chilli flakes		¼ tsp	
vegetable stock (see page 154)	500 ml	16 fl oz	2 cups
canned chopped tomatoes	600 g	1 lb 5 oz	
tomato purée/paste		1 tbsp	
a good squeeze of lemon juice or to taste			
black pepper			
red kidney beans, canned or cooked as per instructions on pack	130 g	4 ½ oz	¾ cup
flageolet beans, canned or cooked as per instructions on pack	130 g	4 ½ oz	¾ cup
sweetcorn, canned, or 1 ear fresh corn, cooked and cut off the cob	130 g	4 ½ oz	¾ cup
FOR THE GARNISH:			
a good handful of roughly chopped fresh coriander/ cilantro leaves and stalks			
a few shavings of pecorino cheese			

Soften the onion in half the olive oil over a medium heat. Add the crushed garlic and the chilli flakes and cook, stirring, for 1 minute. Do not allow the garlic to colour. Add the vegetable stock and the chopped tomatoes, the tomato paste, lemon juice and black pepper. Rinse the beans under running water and add together with the corn to the soup. Bring back to the boil, adding the remaining olive oil, and simmer gently for 20 minutes. Adjust seasoning if necessary. Off the heat and just before serving, add the fresh coriander and the shavings of pecorino.

SERVES 4

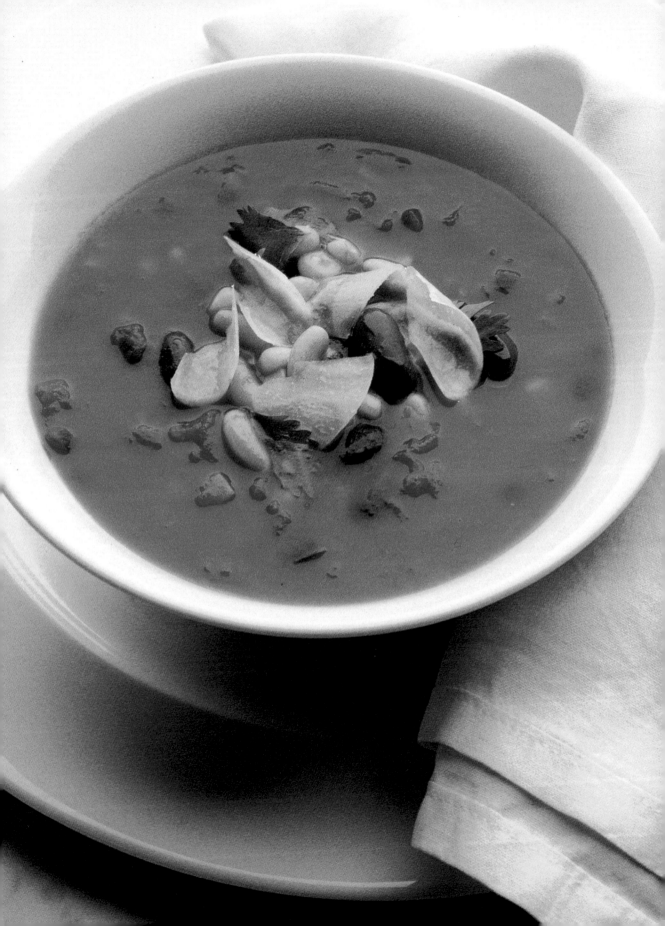

CORN CHOWDER

This is a sweet syrupy soup that is pretty and has a pleasing texture. Use one large ear of fresh corn, simmered for 5 minutes in boiling water and drained. When cool enough to handle, cut down the cob with a sharp knife to remove the niblets. Alternatively, use canned corn.

	METRIC	IMPERIAL	CUPS
sunflower oil		2 tbsp	
sweet onion, roughly chopped	170 g	6 oz	1 cup
celery, roughly chopped, reserve some of the leaves to garnish	115 g	4 oz	1 cup
waxy potatoes with their skins, roughly chopped	140 g	5 oz	1 cup
fresh thyme		1 tbsp	
all-purpose wheat-free flour		2 tbsp	
chicken or vegetable stock (see pages 154 or 155)	500 ml	16 fl oz	2 cups
sheep's or goat's milk	250 ml	8 fl oz	1 cup
plenty of black pepper, (at least 8–10 twists of the mill)			
fresh lemon juice		3 tbsp	
sweetcorn	170 g	6 oz	1 cup

In a heavy pan, heat the oil with the onion and celery and cook over a medium heat for 3 minutes. Add the potato and thyme to the onion mixture, stir and cook for another minute.

Off the heat add the flour and stir in the stock and milk. Return to the heat and bring to the boil, stirring constantly.

Add plenty of black pepper and lemon juice. Add the cup of cooked sweetcorn, cover and simmer over a gentle heat until the potatoes are just tender, about 10 minutes.

SERVES 3

TARAMASALATA

This is simple to make, delicious to eat, and stores well covered in the refrigerator for up to a week. At cooking school we were taught to add all sorts of things to this classic dish including breadcrumbs and olive oil. I like this simple unadulterated recipe the best. Just use equal amounts of goat's cheese and fish roe and, depending upon the saltiness of the smoked roe, add lemon juice to taste. A wonderful source of protein.

	METRIC	IMPERIAL	CUPS
smoked cod's roe (select one that is soft without a thick skin)	250 g	8 ½ oz	
mild goat's cream cheese	250 g	8 ½ oz	
1 clove garlic (optional)			
lemon juice		2 tbsp	

Simply mix together in a bowl or food processor. Serve with blinis, (see page 26), and black olives. Enough for 6 people as a starter, or 4 as a main course for lunch served with a green salad.

SERVES 4–6

DUCK TERRINE WITH GREEN PEPPERCORNS

	METRIC	IMPERIAL	CUPS
½ red onion			
6 cloves garlic			
duck meat	225 g	8 oz	
chicken meat	115 g	4 oz	
1 egg			
ground nutmeg		2 tsp	
ground mixed spice/apple-pie spice		4 tsp	
all-purpose wheat-free flour		2 tbsp	
tomato purée/paste		1 tsp	
mixed dried herbs/Italian seasoning		3 tsp	
black pepper		1 tbsp	
soft green peppercorns (bottled)		1 tbsp	
4 whole duck livers			
1 bay leaf			

Preheat the oven to 180°C/350°F/Gas 4. In a food processor, mince/grind the onion, garlic, duck and chicken meats until smooth. With the motor running add the egg, nutmeg, mixed spice, flour and tomato purée. Blend well. Put this mixture into a bowl and stir in the dried herbs, pepper and peppercorns.

Line a small loaf tin with greaseproof paper/baking parchment. Cut the paper into two strips, arrange one lengthways and the other across the tin. Leave extra length to fold back across the top of the tin when filled. Put half the mixture into the prepared tin then add a layer of duck livers. Put the remaining mixture on top. Tap the bottom of the tin lightly on the work surface to ensure that there are no air pockets and that the corners are filled. Smooth, then arrange the bay leaf on top. Now carefully fold over the overlaps of greaseproof paper to form a parcel. Cover the top with foil and place the tin in a baking dish. Pour boiling water into the baking dish to rise halfway up the tin, and place in the oven for 1½ hours or until the juices run clearly when a skewer is inserted into the centre of the terrine. Remove the foil and allow to cool for 15 minutes. Drain off the juices and weigh down with heavy weights until completely cool. Turn out of the tin. Carefully remove the greaseproof paper and wrap with clingfilm/plastic wrap. Refrigerate for 2–3 days before eating.

Cut 2 thin slices per person. Arrange on a plate with a spoonful of cranberry relish (see page 149).

SERVES 8–10

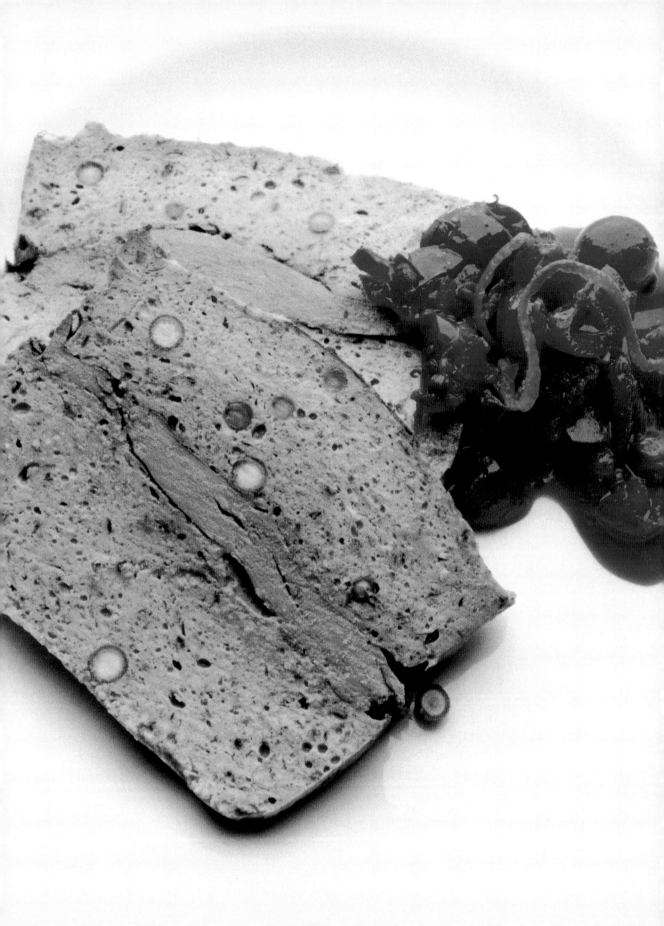

QUICK AND EASY CHICKEN LIVER PATE

Livers from organic chickens are large, firm and healthy. They are included with the giblets accompanying a whole bird and can be made into this quick and easy pâté in a few minutes. The juniper berries are the key ingredient. They impart a hardly discernible sweet, fruity flavour.

	METRIC	IMPERIAL	CUPS
1 large organic chicken liver, chopped			
1 medium red onion, sliced			
2 cloves garlic, crushed			
dried mixed herbs/Italian seasoning		1 tsp	
dried juniper berries (about 10)		1 tsp	
2 dried bay leaves			
hard margarine, depending upon size of liver	115–170 g	4–6 oz	½ –¾ cup

Put all the ingredients in a frying pan and cook over a gentle heat until the onion is soft and the liver has lost its pinkness. Discard the bay leaves, put all the ingredients into a food processor and blend until smooth. Spoon the mixture into a ramekin dish and chill in the refrigerator.

The quantities need not be exact, but aim for roughly the same amount of margarine in weight as the liver. Use a hard margarine, because it will set the pâté when cold.

SERVES 2

PUY LENTILS WITH GINGER

This makes a good vegetarian meal option served with a baked sweet potato. It is excellent served hot or cold with strongly flavoured fish like sardines, blue fish or mackerel, or with grilled chicken.

	METRIC	IMPERIAL	CUPS
Puy lentils, prepared and cooked as per instructions on the pack, or canned lentils which have been rinsed well and drained	400 g	14 oz	2 cups
grated fresh root ginger		1½ – 2 tbsp	
grated garlic		½ tbsp	
olive oil		2 tbsp	
sunflower oil		1 tbsp	
carrot, coarsely grated	140 g	5 oz	1 cup
tomato, chopped, leaving the skin on if organic but removing seeds	260 g	9 oz	1 cup

In a sauté pan, fry the ginger and garlic in the hot oil for 1 minute. Remove from heat and stir in the carrot. The heat remaining in the pan should be enough to cook the carrot in a few seconds. Return the pan to a medium heat and stir-fry the tomatoes and Puy lentils until heated through but not mushy, about 2 minutes.

SERVES 4

BLINIS

	METRIC	IMPERIAL	CUPS
buckwheat flour	55 g	2 oz	scant ½ cup
all purpose wheat-free flour	55 g	2 oz	scant ½ cup
bicarbonate of soda/baking soda		1 tsp	
olive oil		1 tsp	
sunflower oil	30 ml	1 fl oz	2 tbsp
2 small eggs, beaten			
water	150 ml	¼ pt	⅔ cup

Sift the dry ingredients into a bowl. Make a well in the centre. Pour in the oils and eggs and stir, bringing the flour in from the sides. As the mixture thickens, add the water by degrees, stirring with a balloon whisk, until the mixture has the consistency of thick cream. Let stand at room temperature for 15 minutes to allow the liquds to be absorbed by the flour. If mixture has thickened too much, stir in a little water until the desired thickness is achieved. Pour enough mixture for a blini 13 cm/5 in across into a moderately heated griddle. When holes appear on the surface turn and then cook for a very short time on the other side.

The blinis should be thin. If they become too thick either swirl the mixture in the pan to make a thinner pancake, or reduce the thickness of the mixture by adding a small amount of liquid.

The cooked blinis will be golden brown, soft in texture and will keep wrapped in the refrigerator for several days. Warm in a napkin over steam before serving if preferred.

Ideal to serve with various accompaniments including smoked salmon, caviar, chopped hard-boiled egg, chopped spring onions/scallions, aubergine/eggplant pâté, taramasalata (see page 21), all with sheep's yogurt.

MAKES 10–12 BLINIS

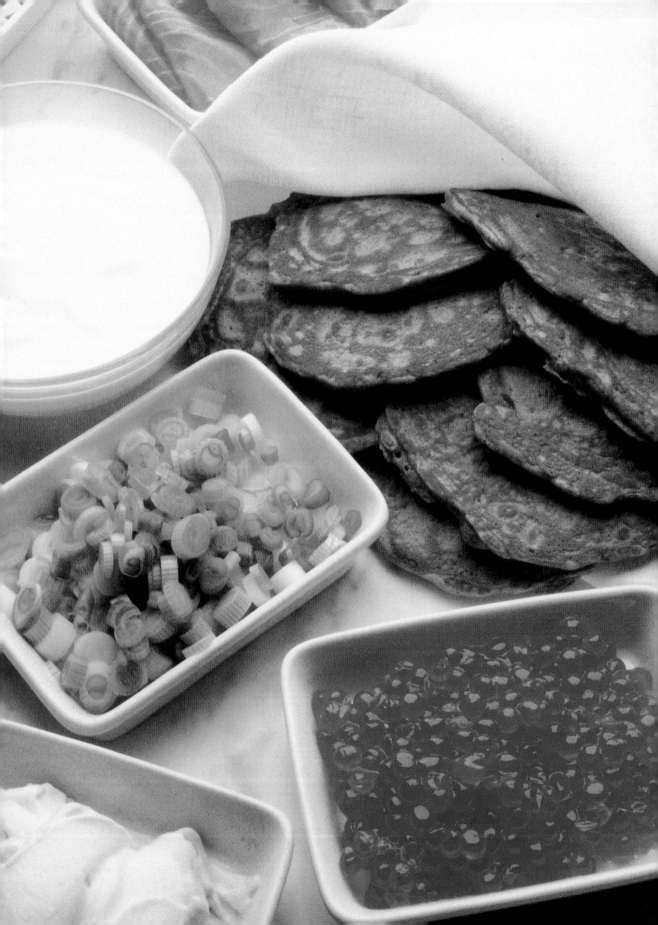

CRISPY CORN FRITTERS

These fritters go well with griddled chicken or duck livers. It is the folded-in egg whites that make these fritters so crispy. I prefer to use fresh corn in season, but canned corn will do almost as well.

	METRIC	IMPERIAL	CUPS
4 duck or chicken livers (optional)			
FOR THE FRITTERS:			
cooked corn niblets or canned corn	200 g	7 oz	1 ¼ cups
all-purpose wheat-free flour		2 tbsp	
1 egg, separated			
goat's milk			
black pepper			
chopped parsley		1 tbsp	
sunflower oil for frying			

Put half the corn into a small bowl and mash with a fork. In a bowl, combine the flour, egg yolk, milk and pepper to form a smooth batter the consistency of single/light cream. Stir in all the corn and the parsley. Whisk the egg white to soft peaks and gently fold into the batter with a large metal spoon. The whites give the fritters the light, crisp texture so be careful not to destroy the air bubbles in the whisked whites.

Heat a shallow amount of oil in a frying pan/skillet and drop 1 tbsp of mixture into the heated oil. When the edges become brown, turn over carefully and cook for a short time on the other side. Remove from the oil and drain thoroughly on kitchen paper. Serve immediately.

If the livers are to be used, dry-fry them in a griddle pan and serve on top of the corn fritters.

MAKES ABOUT 6 FRITTERS

SWISS CHARD GRATIN

Swiss chard is a wonderful vegetable, almost two vegetables in one. The green leaves can be cooked in a similar way to spinach, and the stalks can be prepared separately. The latter have a wonderful flavour which is a cross between celery and asparagus. This recipe uses the entire vegetable and is ideal for finishing up bits of cheese. The leaves 'steam' under the béchamel sauce. Swiss chard grows vigorously, and the outer leaves can become very large with the white stalks growing up to 10 cm/4 in across. Cut very large stalks to form convenient bite-sized pieces. Use a cheese of your choice. I use 45 g / 1 ½ oz / ¼ cup crumbled feta, and 45 g / 1 ½ oz / ½ cup goat's Cheddar, coarsely grated. If you like the flavour of blue cheese, use Roquefort instead of the feta, or a combination of both. Pecorino can also be grated and used with the Cheddar.

	METRIC	IMPERIAL	CUPS
Swiss chard	450 g	1 lb	
a little margarine			
black pepper			
cheese of your choice, grated	90 g	3 oz	¾ cup
classic béchamel sauce (see page 153)			

Preheat the oven to 190°C/375°F/Gas 5.

Wash the Swiss chard thoroughly, discarding any discoloured bits. Pat dry with kitchen paper. Cut the stalks away from the green leaves and cut them into bite-sized pieces. Steam the stalks for 2 minutes. Grease a shallow baking dish with margarine and arrange the stalks in a shallow layer. Grind over black pepper and dot with half the grated cheese. Cut the green leaves into shreds and place in a layer over the stalks. These leaves will be springy but will wilt as soon as you pour over the hot béchamel sauce. Top with the remaining grated cheese. Place in the preheated oven for 35 minutes.

SERVES 4

ROAST AUBERGINE, SWEET POTATO, CHICK-PEAS AND RED PEPPERS WITH SPINACH

	METRIC	IMPERIAL	CUPS
1 medium aubergine/eggplant			
1 red bell pepper			
1 sweet potato			
olive oil			
a pinch of cayenne			
black pepper			
lemon juice		1 tbsp	
canned chick-peas/garbanzo beans, rinsed, or dried chick-peas, prepared following manufacturers' instructions	425 g	15 oz	2¼ cups
paprika		½ tsp	
a little freshly grated nutmeg			
spinach, shredded	55 g	2 oz	1 cup
sheep's yogurt (optional)	225 ml	8 fl oz	1 cup
fresh mint leaves, chopped (optional)			

Preheat the oven to 230°C/450°F/Gas 8. Cut the aubergine into cubes 1 cm/½ in thick, leaving the skin on. Cut the pepper in half and remove the seeds and stalk. Cut it into lengths 6 mm/¼ in wide and cut each strip in half. Peel the sweet potato and cut it into ½ in cubes.

Put the aubergine pieces into a large mixing bowl and add 2 tbsp of the olive oil and stir until the oil is absorbed. Sprinkle over a pinch of cayenne, some black pepper and ½ tbsp lemon juice. Lightly oil a roasting pan and place the aubergine pieces at one end of the tray, one layer deep. Place the cut pepper pieces in a single layer next to the aubergine. Put the sweet potato cubes and chick-peas into a mixing bowl and add ½ tbsp olive oil, the lemon juice, the paprika and a little freshly grated nutmeg. Stir to blend. Place the sweet potato pieces and chick-peas on the roasting tray, scraping out any spices that remain in the mixing bowl with a spatula. Cook in the hot oven for 30 minutes. The vegetables should now be cooked through but firm enough to hold their shape. They should also be slightly charred. Scrape the vegetables up from the tray and toss in the spinach. The spinach will not cook. Add black pepper. This is a 'dry' dish, but if you prefer, add more oil and lemon juice to moisten. Alternatively serve with the yogurt mixed with the mint leaves. This dish may be served hot or cold.

SERVES 4

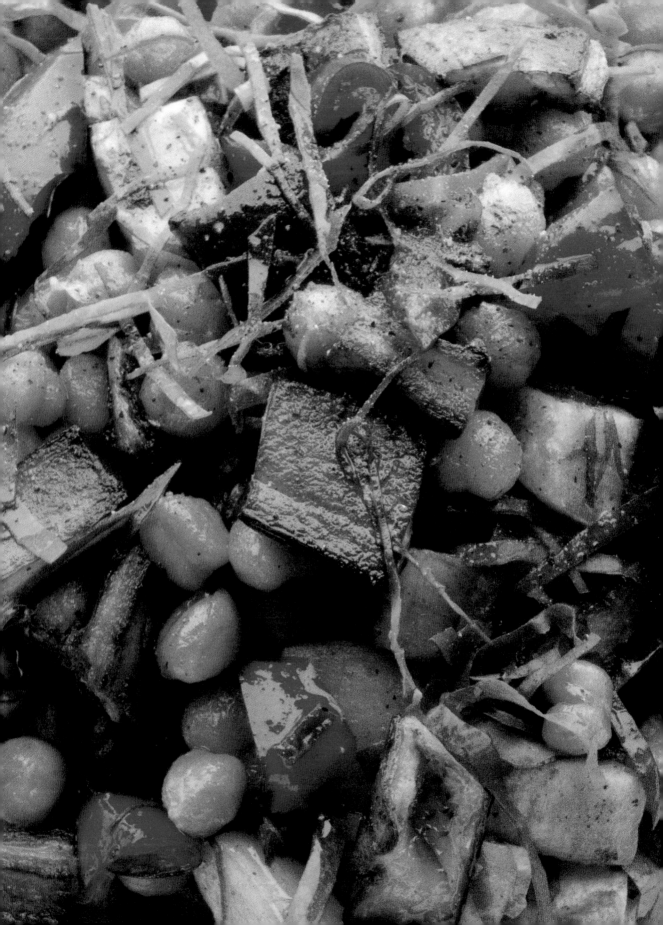

BRAISED RED CABBAGE

The flavour of the cabbage improves when prepared a day or two in advance. It keeps very well in the refrigerator for up to a week and can be reheated when required. It is also good served cold.

	METRIC	IMPERIAL	CUPS
2 red cabbages, sliced			
chopped onion		2 tbsp	
olive oil		5 tbsp	
2 cloves garlic, crushed			
caraway seeds (optional)		2 tbsp	
4 Cox's apples or other sweet apples, peeled, cored and cut into eighths (no need to peel organic apples)			
juice and grated zest of ½ lemon			
black pepper			
balsamic vinegar		1 tbsp	
water			

Cook the onion in the olive oil until soft. Add the garlic and caraway seeds (if using), and cook over high heat for a few seconds until the seeds pop. Add the rest of the ingredients, including about 150 ml/¼ pt/⅔ cup water, cover and cook over a low oven for ¾ hour or until the apples and cabbage are tender. Stir from time to time during the cooking, and add more water if necessary.

SERVES 10

GREEN BEANS WITH CHERRY TOMATOES

Maurice More-Betty was a well-known cookery writer and TV chef. He also ran a cooking school out of his duplex in the Upper East Side. When we moved to New York with our young family, we lived in what had been Maurice's apartment and thus inherited his splendid kitchen. Our paths crossed again in Shelter Island where we both had homes. Maurice was extremely kind to the girls, and his invitations to lunch were a great treat. He had noticed Lucy's eczema and had rightly surmised that the store-bought ice cream that Lucy ate with her friends was contributing to the problem. He made tubs of wonderful sorbet especially for Lucy, made from the fresh peaches grown locally.

I remember one lunch-time in particular. The weather was exceptionally clear and from Maurice's house, perched high on a bluff, we could see across Peconic Bay, over the North Fork of Long Island and all the way to the Connecticut Sound. Maurice served us a simple chicken dish, similar to the one described on page 99 and these beans. For the girls, the lunch is memorable because Maurice's dog Oscar was stung by a hornet.

	METRIC	IMPERIAL	CUPS
green beans	225 g	8 oz	
cherry tomatoes	170 g	6 oz	
sweet onion	115 g	4 oz	²/₃ cup
olive oil		2 tbsp	
1 large clove garlic, crushed			
black pepper			
lemon juice			

Top and tail the beans and cut into pieces 5 cm/2 in long. Steam for 3–4 minutes, leaving the beans quite crunchy.

Cut the cherry tomatoes in halves. Finely chop the onion and fry it in the olive oil until soft and golden brown. Add the garlic and cook for 1 minute. Stir the steamed beans and the tomato halves into the onion mixture for a couple of minutes until they are heated through, but the tomatoes still retain their shape. Gently stir so that all the vegetables are mixed and coated with the oil, onion and garlic mixture. Season to taste with black pepper and a squeeze of lemon juice.

This dish can be served hot or cold.

SERVES 4

MIXED VEGETABLE CURRY

Serve this with rice as a main course or as an accompaniment to Chicken with Coconut Cream and Aromatic Spices (see page 98). For the pound of vegetables I would suggest using cauliflower florets and sliced stalk, green beans cut into 5 cm/2 in pieces, large carrot cut into 1.25 cm / ½ in chunks and 75 g/3 oz/½ cup peas. Potato pieces, chick-peas, okra etc can also be included.

	METRIC	IMPERIAL	CUPS
1 medium onion, chopped			
vegetable oil		4 tbsp	
8 cardamom pods			
coriander seeds		1 tsp	
cumin seeds		1 tsp	
curry powder		1 tsp	
turmeric		½ tsp	
black pepper			
a variety of mixed vegetables	450 g	1 lb	
4 tomatoes, chopped			
water	150 ml	¼ pint	⅔ cup
sheep's or goat's yogurt or juice of ¼ lemon (optional)		1 tbsp	

Soften the onion in oil. Add the cardamom and all the seeds, and fry for a couple of minutes. Add curry powder, turmeric and black pepper and fry for another minute. Stir in the vegetables, chopped tomatoes and water. Cover and cook until the vegetables are just tender (more or less liquid can be used depending on the desired dryness of the curry). Stir in yogurt or lemon juice (if using).

SERVES 4

MUSHROOM AND MOREL SOUP

The delicious, subtle flavour of the morels combined with the tanginess of the yoghurt and coriander make this soup special enough for a party.

	METRIC	IMPERIAL	CUPS
olive oil		2 tbsp	
1 small onion, roughly chopped			
1 large potato (skin left on if organic), cut into chunks			
organic white button mushrooms including their stalks, roughly chopped	225 g	8 oz	3 cups (whole)
Dijon mustard		1 tsp	
black pepper to taste			
dry white wine	100 ml	3½ fl oz	½ cup
good chicken or vegetable stock	350 ml	12 fl oz	1½ cups
1 pack dried morel mushrooms (about 15)	20 g	¾ oz	1½ cups
sheep's yoghurt		1 heaped tbsp	
a few sprigs of fresh coriander/cilantro			

Soak the morels in 350 ml/12 fl oz/1½ cups warm water for about 20 minutes, then drain, reserving the soaking liquid. Chop the morels coarsely.

Heat the oil in a large saucepan. Add the onion and sweat for about 4 minutes until soft but not browned. Add the potato and button mushrooms to the pan and stir to combine. Add the mustard, pepper and wine and boil rapidly to reduce the liquid by half.

Add the stock and morel soaking liquid and cover and simmer for 20 minutes or until the potato is tender.

Put the soup in a blender or food processor and liquidize until smooth. Return soup to the pan, straining it through a sieve, if desired. Add the chopped morels and simmer gently for 5 minutes to impart their flavour to the soup.

Ladle soup into two bowls, add a spoonful of yoghurt to the centre of each and garnish with coriander.

SERVES 2

SALMON TARTARE WITH JAPANESE GINGER

My twin sister, Anne, has two delicious salmon recipes using Japanese pickled ginger. (See also Roasted Salmon with Sultanas and Japanese Ginger, page 74.) The ginger is pink and finely sliced and available in some supermarkets and speciality stores. This is a quick and easy party dish.

	METRIC	IMPERIAL	CUPS
salmon tail fillet, boned but with the skin left on	350 g	12 oz	
Japanese pickled ginger		2 tbsp	
FOR THE MARINADE:			
olive oil		2 tbsp	
good tamari		4 tbsp	
balsamic vinegar		2 tbsp	
5 spring onions/scallions, finely sliced			
juice from the ginger		4 tbsp	
black pepper			
wasabi (Japanese horseradish) or		¼ tsp	
Dijon mustard (optional)		1 tsp	

Mix the marinade ingredients together and pour over the fish, skin side down, so that the onions cover the top of the flesh. Then turn the fish over carefully so that the skin side is up but the onions are under the fillet. Cover with clingfilm/plastic wrap and marinate for 1 hour.

Slice thinly, horizontally, holding the tail end firmly in your left hand. If you prefer, the fish may be cut into small cubes or strips. Arrange the slices (or strips) on plates, and spoon over a little of the marinade. Sprinkle over some of the onion and the chopped pickled ginger.

Any leftovers can be marinated for 24 hours, in which case do not spoon over any more marinade, just sprinkle over a little of the onion and the pickled ginger.

Garnish with lamb's lettuce/corn salad, frisée or watercress.

SERVES 6

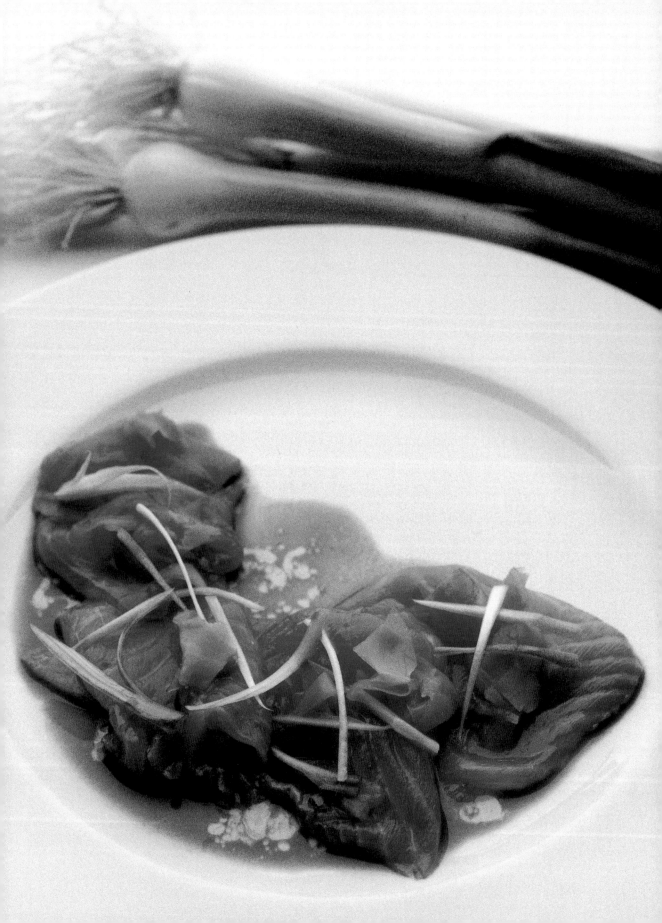

INDIVIDUAL MUSHROOM SOUFFLÉS

These 'soufflés' are made without flour or whisked egg whites, so they do not rise as much as the Cheese and Garlic Soufflé (see page 58). They are extremely simple to make and are good as a starter or as a light lunch dish served with salad.

	METRIC	IMPERIAL	CUPS
brown or button mushrooms	200 g	7 oz	3 cups
goat's cream cheese	150 g	5 ½ oz	
1 clove garlic			
2 slices sweet onion			
3 eggs			
pecorino cheese, finely grated (retain 1 tbsp for garnish)	55 g	2 oz	½ cup
chopped fresh chives, plus a little extra for garnish		1 tbsp	
a little black pepper			
vegetable oil			

Preheat the oven to 200°C/400°F/Gas 6. Retain one of the mushrooms for garnish. In a food processor using the blade, blend the mushrooms, cream cheese, garlic, onion and eggs until the mixture is smooth. Stir in the pecorino, chives and black pepper.

Lightly oil 6 ramekin dishes with vegetable oil. Divide the mixture between the dishes, sprinkle the top with the remaining grated pecorino cheese and decorate with a thin slice of mushroom on top.

Bake in the preheated hot oven for 18 minutes or until risen, golden and just firm to the touch. Sprinkle over a few chopped chives and serve immediately.

SERVES 6

POTATO GRATIN

This is the French classic but made using goat's milk and cheese and substituting cream and butter with yogurt and margarine. The result tastes delicious and remarkably authentic. The exact amount of liquid needed will depend upon the type of potatoes used. Some absorb more liquid than others. I prefer to use waxy potatoes because the slices remain separate, and they do not absorb much liquid. Check the potatoes halfway through the cooking time and if they have dried up, add another 100 ml/3 $\frac{1}{2}$ fl oz/$\frac{1}{2}$ cup goat's milk.

	METRIC	IMPERIAL	CUPS
potatoes, not peeled	450 g	1 lb	
margarine			
goat's milk	125 ml	4 fl oz	$\frac{1}{2}$ cup
black pepper			
freshly grated nutmeg			
1 small clove garlic, crushed			
sheep's yogurt	80 ml	2 $\frac{3}{4}$ fl oz	$\frac{1}{3}$ cup
cornflour/cornstarch		$\frac{1}{2}$ tbsp	
goat's Cheddar cheese, grated	90 g	3 oz	$\frac{3}{4}$ cup

Preheat the oven to 200°C/400°F/Gas 6. Liberally grease a shallow ovenproof serving dish with margarine.

Slice the potatoes finely and put half the slices in a layer in the dish. Use any small or misshapen slices for this layer and retain the best slices for the top layer. Pour over 60 ml/2 fl oz/$\frac{1}{4}$ cup of the goat's milk, and sprinkle with the black pepper, nutmeg, and crushed garlic. Dot with a little margarine. Mix the yogurt with the cornflour and spread this over. Finish with half the cheese. Arrange the rest of the potato slices in a layer, neatly overlapping each other. Pour over the remaining milk. Sprinkle with black pepper and nutmeg and the remaining cheese. Dot with a little margarine and cook in the oven for 45 minutes or until the top is golden and the potatoes are tender but not mushy.

SERVES 4

BROAD BEANS, PEAS, ASPARAGUS AND SPRING ONIONS WITH MINT

I visited Spain for the first time when I was pregnant with our eldest daughter, Poppy. Like most women in this condition, food took on a new meaning. I felt extremely fit and had a good appetite, but very few types of foods appealed to me. It was springtime and this dish, made using all the available new season's vegetables, was one that I particularly enjoyed.

	METRIC	IMPERIAL	CUPS
shelled broad/fava beans	450 g	1 lb	3 cups
shelled peas	200 g	7 oz	1 ½ cups
sugar peas in their pods	200 g	7 oz	
asparagus, washed	300 g	10 ½ oz	
spring onions/scallions	300 g	10 ½ oz	
olive oil	80 ml	2 ¾ fl oz	⅓ cup
2 large cloves garlic, crushed			
fresh mint leaves, chopped	15 g	½ oz	½ cup
black pepper			
lemon juice			
a little lemon zest (optional)			

Steam the broad beans until just tender. This will depend on the size and age of the beans, so keep an eye on them. Steam the peas and sugar peas for a couple of minutes until just tender. If the asparagus is very young and the spears are small, leave them whole. If larger spears are used, cut these into pieces 5 cm/2 in long. Steam as before. Cut the white bulb part of the spring onions into lengths about 7.5 cm/3 in long. Cut the green part into slices and put to one side.

Put the olive oil into a large sauté pan over a moderate heat and cook the white parts of the spring onions for a couple of minutes. This will depend upon the size of the vegetables, so as before, do not overcook. Just as they are beginning to soften add the crushed garlic, stir into the oil and cook for a minute. Tip in the steamed beans, peas, asparagus and sugar peas and toss in the oil so that all the vegetables are thoroughly coated. Add a little more oil to moisten, if necessary.

At the last minute stir in the sliced green part of the onions, the mint and the seasonings to taste. Serve hot or cold on its own, or as one of a selection of dishes to make up a main course.

SERVES 4

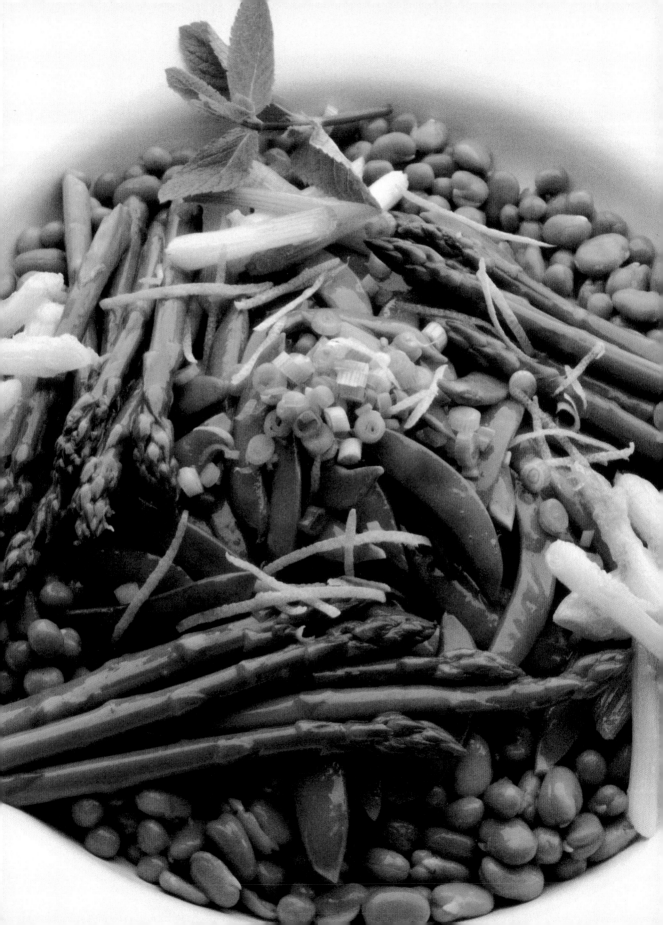

ROASTED PLUM TOMATOES

4 large ripe plum tomatoes

olive oil

1 clove garlic

black pepper

Preheat the oven to its hottest setting. Brush an ovenproof dish with a little olive oil. Cut the tomatoes in half lengthways. Peel and cut the garlic into fine garlic shards. Place the tomatoes, cut side up, in the oiled dish and pierce with the shards of garlic. Use at least 2 shards per tomato half. Brush with olive oil and dust with freshly ground black pepper. Cook on the top shelf of the oven for 15–20 minutes. They should be cooked through but not collapsed. Finish under the grill/broiler to char slightly if preferred.

SERVES 4

PARSNIP AND GARLIC MASH

This is a sweet tasting and flavourful mash, which is delicious with grilled/broiled chicken sausages.

	METRIC	IMPERIAL	CUPS
1 large potato, cut into chunks			
1 large parsnip, cut into chunks			
olive oil		3 tbsp	
8 spring onions/scallions, including the green parts, finely sliced			
2 large cloves of garlic crushed			
a good pinch of mace			
black pepper to taste			

Cook potato and parsnip together in a large pan of boiling water until soft. Drain.

Heat oil in a large saucepan and quickly sauté the spring onions and garlic. Add the drained parsnip and potato and mash. Season with mace and black pepper. Serve piping hot.

SERVES 4

CHICORY, APPLE, TOMATO AND ROQUEFORT SALAD

This is a versatile salad. For a variation, try using chopped cooked beetroot instead of the tomatoes. The beetroots should be tossed in olive oil separately to avoid their juice colouring the other ingredients. Walnuts or toasted pumpkin seeds can be used instead of the cheese.

	METRIC	IMPERIAL	CUPS
4 heads chicory/endives, sliced			
4 apples, chopped (unpeeled if organic)			
chopped tomatoes in equal amounts to apples			
Roquefort cheese, crumbled	115 g	4 oz	generous ½ cup
seasoning and herbs to taste (e.g. chopped parsley, pepper and lemon juice)			

Mix all ingredients together in a bowl. No dressing is needed for this delicious refreshing salad, but it must be assembled at the last minute otherwise the apples will discolour.

SERVES 4

WATERCRESS AND ORANGE SALAD

	METRIC	IMPERIAL	CUPS
2 large bunches watercress, washed			
2 oranges, peled and segmented			
toasted sesame seeds		1 tbsp	

Chop the stalks of the watercress into 2.5cm/1 in long pieces and place with the leaves in a bowl with the orange segments. Mix. Sprinkle over the sesame seeds.

SERVES 4

CORN, TOMATO, RED ONION AND AVOCADO SALAD

	METRIC	IMPERIAL	CUPS
chopped tomatoes	500 g	1 lb 2 oz	2 cups
cooked sweetcorn	300 g	10 ½ oz	2 cups
finely chopped red onion		3 ½ tbsp	
zest of 2 limes			
juice of 1 lime, or more to taste			
plenty of black pepper			
1 avocado, diced			
1 bunch fresh coriander/cilantro leaves			

Mix all the ingredients in a bowl with the exception of the avocado and coriander which should be added just before serving. Scissor the coriander roughly into the salad mix.

SERVES 4

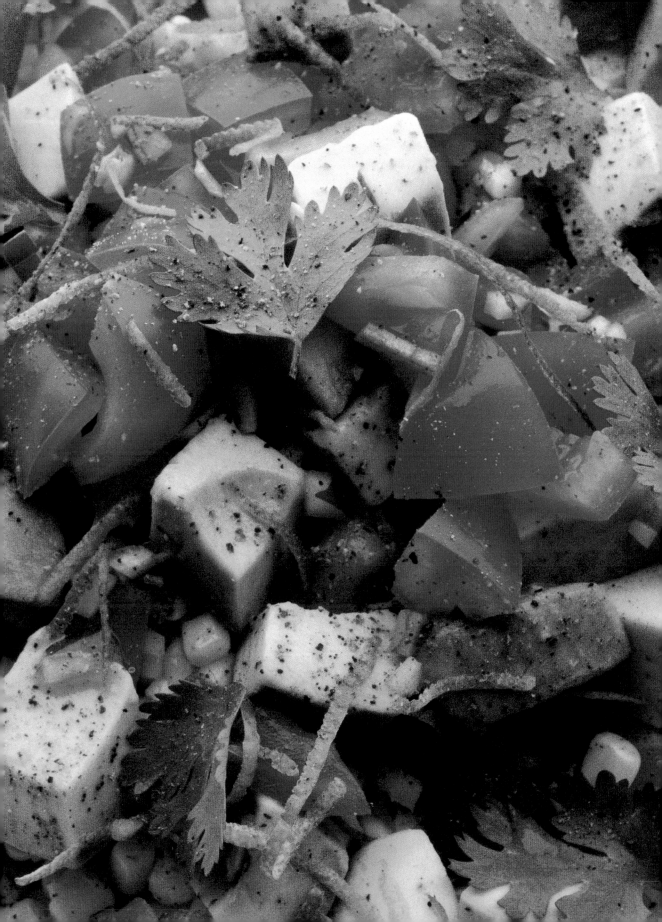

BLACK BEAN AND FENNEL SALAD

This is a nourishing but refreshing salad with a pretty, rosy hue. It is good with grilled/broiled oily fish such as blue fish, mackerel or sardines. Or just add 450g/1lb/2 cups of crumbled ricotta for a complete vegetarian meal.

Be careful when you work with the chilli. Use gloves and wash your hands thoroughly afterwards as chilli seeds can burn the skin.

	METRIC	IMPERIAL	CUPS
black beans cooked as per instructions on the packet, or canned beans, rinsed thoroughly and drained	350 g	12 oz	2 cups
red onion, finely sliced	90 g	3 oz	½ cup
tomato, seeded and diced	250 g	8 ½ oz	1 cup
fennel bulb, roughly chopped, including the feathery green leaves	140 g	5 oz	1 cup
ricotta cheese, crumbled (optional)	450 g	1 lb	2 cups
FOR THE DRESSING:			
1 hot red chilli, seeded and finely chopped			
grated zest of 1 lemon			
lemon juice		2 tbsp	
olive oil		½ tbsp	
lots of freshly milled black pepper			
finely chopped fresh dill		2 tbsp	

In a small bowl, mix the dressing ingredients, except for the dill, leave to stand for 5 minutes to allow the chillies to flavour the mixture.

Mix the beans, onion, tomato and fennel in a bowl, then stir in the dressing.

Add the dill and ricotta (if desired) just before serving.

SERVES 4

GREEN SALAD

An almost infinite variety of green leaves, herbs, sprouts and vegetables can be used. Choose a combination that gives a good mix of different textures and flavours. Here are some suggestions.

	METRIC	IMPERIAL	CUPS
1 celery heart or fennel bulb, sliced			
1 bunch watercress with the stalks, cut into 2.5 cm/1 in pieces			
1 avocado, chopped in largish pieces			
6 large basil leaves, torn into pieces			
toasted pumpkin seeds (optional)			
any sprouting beans (see page 63)			
any variety of lettuces available and in season			
FOR THE DRESSING:			
Dijon mustard		1 tsp	
balsamic vinegar		1 tbsp	
olive oil		3 tbsp	

Put the salad ingredients into a bowl and toss with the dressing. This salad has a pleasing variety of textures and tastes. It is robust enough to serve as a 'vegetable' and is excellent with grilled/broiled fish or game.

For a main lunch course, increase the quantities and add toasted seeds, sprouts, nuts or cheese.

SERVES 4

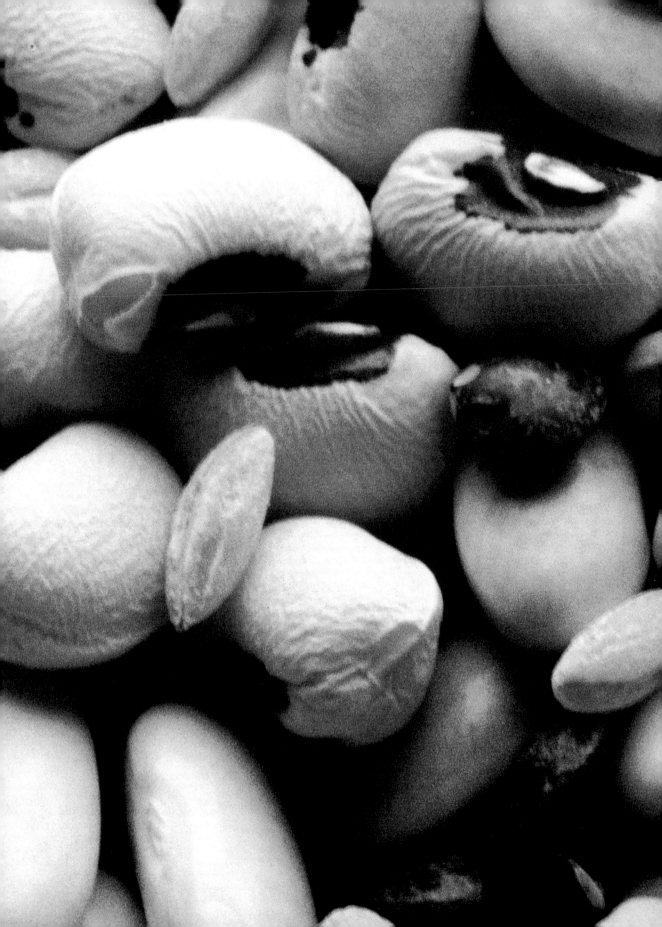

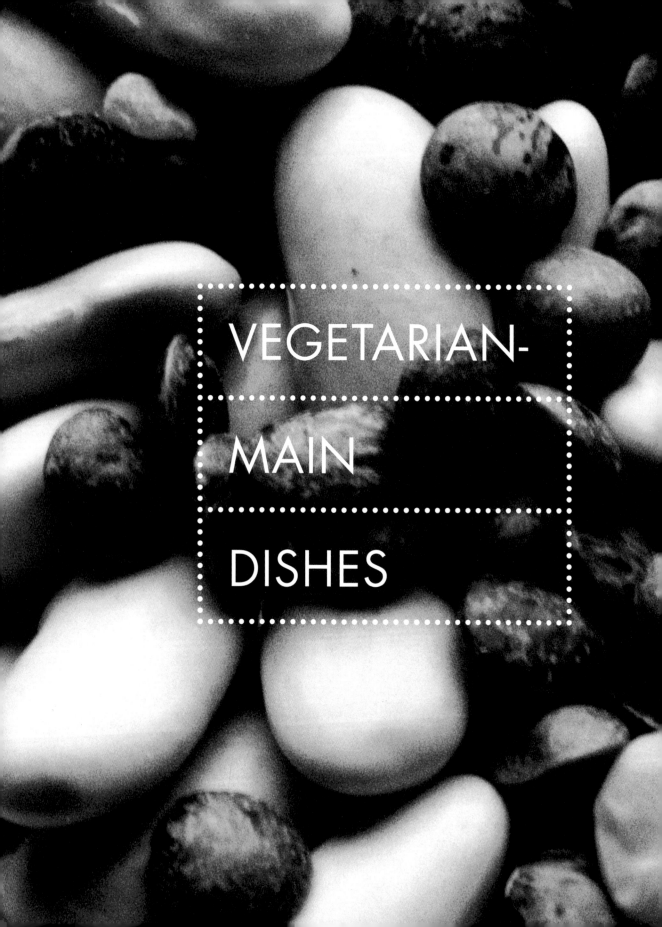

VEGETARIAN-MAIN DISHES

VEGETARIAN CHILLI

This classic dish can be prepared a day in advance.

	METRIC	IMPERIAL	CUPS
½ sweet white onion, finely chopped			
½ red onion, finely chopped			
1 jalapeño pepper, seeded and finely chopped (see page 46)			
¼ red bell pepper, seeded and chopped			
olive oil		6 tbsp	
red chilli flakes		¼ tsp	
ground cinnamon		¼ tsp	
cumin seeds		½ tsp	
dried thyme		½ tsp	
2–3 cloves garlic, crushed			
canned red kidney beans, drained and rinsed under running cold water	175 g	6 oz	1 cup
canned cannelli beans, drained and rinsed under running cold water	175 g	6 oz	1 cup
Puy lentils, cooked according to instructions on pack, or canned lentils, rinsed and drained	200 g	7oz	1 cup
canned tomatoes with their juice	250 g	8½ oz	1 cup
tomato purée/paste		1 tbsp	
fresh chopped flat parsley	55 g	2 oz	1 cup
grated pecorino cheese (optional)			

Soften the onions, jalapeño pepper and red pepper in 4 tbsp of the oil for 4 minutes. Add the chilli flakes, cinnamon, cumin and thyme and cook over high heat for 1 minute. Reduce the heat to medium and add the garlic, beans and lentils. Stir into the mixture and cook for a couple of minutes. Add the tomatoes, tomato purée and remaining olive oil, cover and simmer over a low heat for 15 minutes. Add the parsley just before serving. Serve on its own or with rice. Sprinkle with pecorino if used.

SERVES 3

PENNE GRATIN

A variety of wheat-free pasta is now available from healthfood stores, so select your favourite. We always choose fresh, organic pasta, which has an authentic 'bite'.

	METRIC	IMPERIAL	CUPS
fresh wheat-free penne (or other pasta)	250 g	8½ oz	
sunflower oil		3 tbsp	
Dijon mustard		4 tsp	
plenty of freshly ground black pepper			
½ nutmeg, finely grated			
all-purpose wheat-free flour		3 tbsp	
milk (goat's, sheep's or soya)	500 ml	16 fl oz	2 cups
sheep's Cheddar cheese, grated	115 g	4 oz	1 cup
pecorino, grated	55 g	2 oz	⅔ cup
fresh chives, snipped	15 g	½ oz	1½ cups

Cook the penne as per the instructions on the pack, making sure that it is *al dente*, as it will continue to cook in the sauce when the dish is grilled. Drain.

Put the oil, mustard, pepper, nutmeg and flour into a saucepan and mix together. Add the milk and cook over a gentle heat, stirring until boiling and thickened. Reduce the heat and simmer gently for 3-4 minutes.

Mix the two cheeses together. Take the sauce off the heat and beat in half the cheese until melted. Stir in the penne and chives and mix well. Adjust seasoning to taste.

Lightly grease a shallow ovenproof dish, pour in the mixture and smooth the top. Sprinkle with the remaining cheese and place under a preheated grill/broiler until golden brown. Serve immediately.

SERVES 4

BUCKWHEAT KASHA SALAD WITH HALLOUMI CHEESE

Buckwheat is used extensively in Russian cuisine (see the recipe for Blinis on page 26). Buckwheat contains more than 13 per cent protein and has a high amino acid content. Toasted and cooked like this it adds a nutty taste to any dish. Halloumi is a traditional white, semi-hard sheep's milk cheese.

	METRIC	IMPERIAL	CUPS
1 halloumi cheese			
a little all-purpose wheat-free flour for dusting			
FOR THE KASHA SALAD:			
buckwheat	225g	8oz	2 cups
olive oil		4 tbsp	
water	1 litre	1 ¾ pt	4 cups
mint, finely chopped	55 g	2 oz	1 cup
flat parsley, chopped	55 g	2 oz	1 cup
finely sliced spring onion/scallion		4 tbsp	
cucumber, peeled, seeded and diced	300 g	10 ½ oz	3 cups
lemon juice		4 tbsp	
black pepper			
pumpkin seeds	75 g	3 oz	½ cup

Rinse the buckwheat in plenty of cold running water. Drain thoroughly. Put half the olive oil in a saucepan, add the buckwheat and fry, stirring until toasted and golden. Be careful not to burn. Pour in the water, cover and simmer gently until all the liquid is absorbed. Turn off the heat and leave to stand, covered, for 5 minutes. If there is sediment on the grains, rinse again under running water.

Put the remaining ingredients except the pumpkin seeds in a bowl and mix well. Leave to stand.

Heat a heavy non-stick frying pan/skillet. Do not add any oil. When hot put in the pumpkin seeds and shake over a high heat until the seeds start to 'pop'. Remove from the pan and put on a plate. Sprinkle these over the kasha salad just before serving.

Slice the cheese lengthways to a thickness of about 1 cm/½ in, dust with a little flour and dry-fry in a non-stick pan until the cheese is a rich caramel brown. Serve with the kasha salad.

SERVES 4 as a main meal

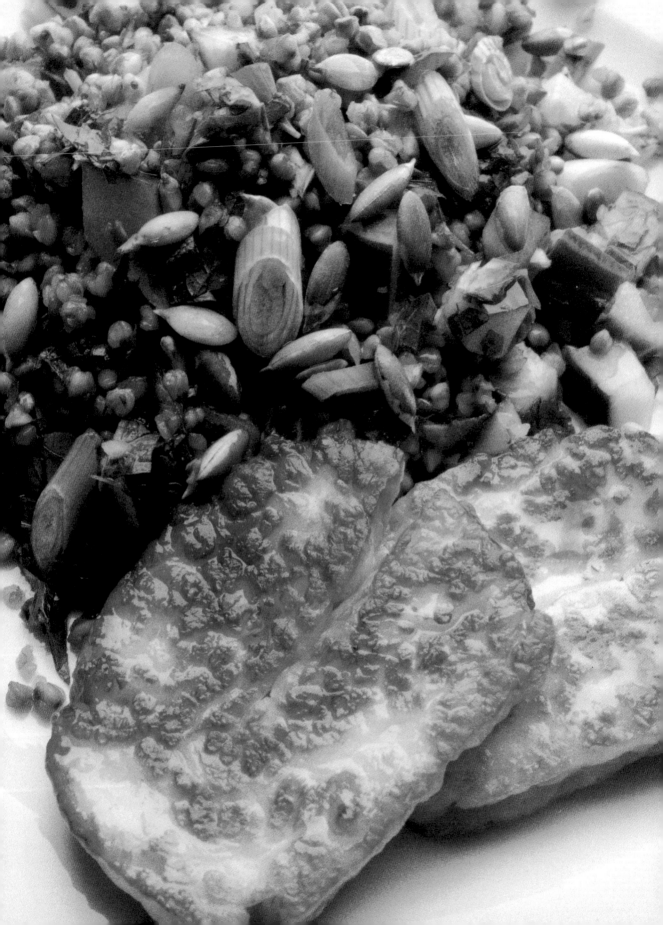

RED CAMARGUE RICE AND ROAST VEGETABLES WITH EGGS

A very colourful red wild rice grows in the Camargue region of France. Brown rice or any other rice of your choice can be used in its place.

	METRIC	IMPERIAL	CUPS
4 hard-boiled eggs			
FOR THE RICE:			
red Camargue rice	200 g	7 oz	generous 1 cup
2 large cloves garlic, peeled and cut in half			
3 bay leaves			
1 sprig fresh rosemary			
olive oil		1 tbsp	
FOR THE DRESSING:			
Dijon mustard		½ tbsp	
lemon juice		1 tsp	
plenty of black pepper			
olive oil		1 tbsp	
chopped fresh parsley		2 tbsp	
chopped fresh basil		4 tbsp	
FOR THE ROAST VEGETABLES:			
1 aubergine/eggplant	300 g	10½ oz	
olive oil			
lemon juice		½ tbsp	
cayenne pepper		⅛ tsp	
black pepper			
2 large courgettes/zucchini	350 g	12 oz	
2 onions	250 g	8½ oz	
2 red sweet bell peppers	200 g	7 oz	

Preheat the oven to its highest setting. Lightly oil a large roasting tray.

Cut the aubergine into slices 2.5 cm/1 in thick and cut these slices into strips 2.5 cm/1 in wide. Cut the strips into batons 5 cm/2 in long. Place in a large bowl. In a small bowl mix 4 tbsp of the olive oil, the lemon juice, cayenne and black pepper. Pour the oil mixture over the aubergine and toss well until it is all absorbed. Place on the roasting tray.

Cut the courgettes in thick slices diagonally and toss in 1 tbsp olive oil and some black pepper. Place on the roasting tray.

Peel the onions and slice in half. Cut each half into 4 pieces through the root end. Toss in ½ tbsp olive oil and place on the roasting tray.

Cut the peppers in half and remove the seeds. Cut into thick strips and cut these strips in half. Place on the roasting tray.

Roast the vegetables in the hot oven for 35–40 minutes until cooked and slightly charred, but retaining their shape.

Cook the rice according to the instructions on the packet, adding the garlic, bay leaves, rosemary and 1 tbsp olive oil to the water. Once the cooking time has been reached, remove from the heat, cover and let stand for 5 minutes. Remove the garlic, bay leaves and rosemary twig.

In a large bowl, mix the dressing ingredients together. Add the cooked rice. Chop the egg whites, add, and mix all these ingredients thoroughly. Adjust seasoning to taste.

Arrange the rice mixture in a serving dish. Put the roast vegetables on top. Push the hard-boiled egg yolks through a fine plastic sieve over the top of the vegetables.

Serve hot or cold.

SERVES 4

THREE ONION RISOTTO

Do not be put off by the quantity of onions necessary for this recipe. The finished dish is surprisingly sweet and colourful and not overwhelmingly 'oniony'.

	METRIC	IMPERIAL	CUPS
3 red onions (weight when peeled and sliced)	375 g	13 oz	2 ¼ cups
2 sweet onions (weight when peeled and chopped)	375 g	13 oz	2 ¼ cups
olive oil	80 ml	2 ¾ fl oz	⅓ cup
6 spring onions	100 g	3 ½ oz	
risotto rice	300 g	10 ½ oz	1 ½ cups
lemon juice	60 ml	2 fl oz	scant ¼ cup
vegetable stock (see page 154)	800 ml	27 fl oz	3 ⅜ cups
plenty of black pepper			
grated pecorino cheese			

Slice the red onions 5 mm/¼ in thick and separate the rings. Roughly chop the sweet onions. Put the red and sweet onions into a heavy saucepan with the olive oil. Cook over a moderate heat, stirring, for 4 minutes.

Cut the bulb part of the spring onions into 5 cm/2 in long pieces. Slice the green parts and set aside. Add the spring onion bulb pieces to the onion mixture and cook, stirring for 1 minute.

Add the rice, cook and stir for 2 minutes over heat to coat thoroughly with the oil. Add the lemon juice and boil away rapidly, stirring. Add the stock by degrees, bring to the boil and simmer gently, stirring. Add black pepper and more stock as it is absorbed by the rice. When adding the final 200 ml/ 7 fl oz/scant 1 cup stock, stir in 55 g/2 oz/½ cup of finely grated pecorino and the sliced spring onion tops. Stir, remove from the heat and let stand, covered, for 5 minutes. Adjust seasoning to taste, then serve with additional grated pecorino cheese.

SERVES 4

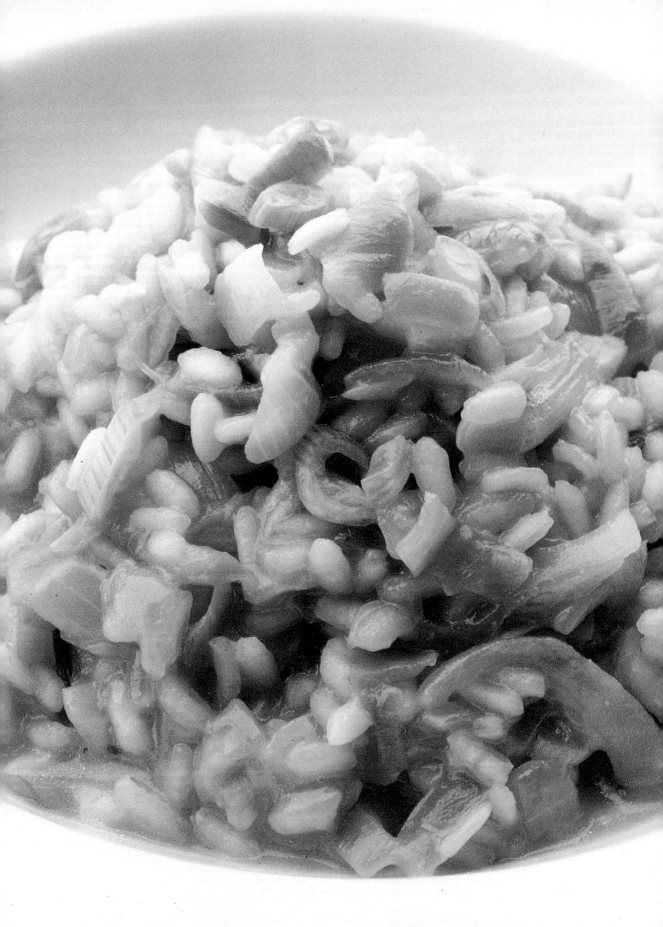

CHEESE AND GARLIC SOUFFLÉ

This recipe is not complicated and the results are well worth the effort.

	METRIC	IMPERIAL	CUPS
sunflower oil		5 tbsp	
olive oil	80 ml	2 ¾ fl oz	⅓ cup
Dijon mustard		1 ½ tsp	
sweet paprika		½ tsp	
hot chilli flakes		¼ tsp	
1 large or 2 small cloves garlic, crushed			
all-purpose wheat-free flour	85 g	2 ¼ oz	⅔ cup
goat's or sheep's milk	500 ml	16 fl oz	2 cups
black pepper			
5 large eggs, separated			
goat's Cheddar cheese, grated	125 g	4 ½ oz	generous 1 cup
pecorino cheese, grated	30 g	1 oz	¼ cup

Preheat the oven to 220°C/425°F/Gas 7.

Put the oils, mustard, paprika, chilli flakes and garlic into a heavy-based saucepan and heat over medium heat for 1 minute. Off the heat stir in the flour. Gradually add the milk, stirring until smooth. Return to the heat and stir until the mixture thickens and boils. Remove from the heat and allow to cool slightly. Add plenty of black pepper and stir in the egg yolks one at a time. Do not overbeat; the mixture will be thick, smooth and glossy. Now lightly mix in the cheeses and set aside while you whisk the egg whites to soft peaks in a dry bowl.

It is the whites that expand during cooking and make the soufflé rise, so it is important to fold them in gently. First stir in 1 tbsp of the egg whites to soften the mixture and make it easier to fold in the remaining whites. Do this a third at a time with a large metal spoon.

Pour the mixture into a lightly oiled 2.25 litre/4 pt/2 qt soufflé dish and bake in the centre of the preheated hot oven for 25–30 minutes or until the mixture has risen and is just firm to the touch.

SERVES 4

SPINACH TART

This classic tart can be served hot or at room temperature. It is good for picnics and lunch boxes.

	METRIC	IMPERIAL	CUPS
1 red onion, sliced			
olive oil		2 tbsp	
2 cloves garlic, crushed			
leaf spinach	400 g	14 oz	
Pastry (see page 155)	500 g	1 lb 2 oz	
5 eggs			
grated pecorino cheese		3 tbsp	
crumbly goat's cheese	200 g	7 oz	
plenty of black pepper			
⅓ fresh nutmeg, grated			

Cook the onion in the oil until just tender. Add the crushed garlic and cook for 1–2 minutes, being careful not to burn as this makes garlic taste bitter.

Steam the spinach then drain. Squeeze out excess moisture (this can be retained as a base for vegetable stock, see page 154) and roughly chop. Place in a large mixing bowl and mix thoroughly with the onion mixture.

Roll out the pastry/dough on a lightly floured surface and use to line a 30 cm/12 in tart tin (preferably with a detachable base). With a fork, lightly make holes in the base and refrigerate for 15 minutes while the oven is warming to 190°C/375°/Gas 5. Bake the pastry case blind for 15 minutes.

Place the eggs, cheeses and seasonings in a bowl and blend thoroughly. Add this to the spinach mixture, and put the filling into the pastry case.

Reduce the heat of the oven to 180°C/350°F/Gas 4 and bake the tart for 30 minutes or until risen, golden and firm to touch.

SERVES 6 as a main course with Three Tomato Salad

SERVES 8 as a starter/appetizer

CELERIAC AND LEEK FRITTATA

This slices well when cold and is a very useful picnic or lunch-box snack. It is equally good if you substitute potato or parsnip for the celeriac.

	METRIC	IMPERIAL	CUPS
celeriac/celery root (weight when peeled)	375 g	13 oz	
good squeeze of lemon juice			
leeks	250 g	8 ½ oz	
sunflower oil		1 tbsp	
hard cheese	150 g	5 ½ oz	
6 large eggs			
chopped fresh dill		4 tbsp	
plenty of black pepper			
grainy mustard		½ tsp	

Peel the celeriac and cut into quarters. Squeeze some lemon juice into a pan of water and bring to the boil. When the water is boiling, add the celeriac and cook until just tender, about 15 minutes.

Meanwhile, wash the leeks and cut into thick slices. Put the oil into a non-stick omelette pan and fry the leeks quickly over a high heat until just softening and starting to brown slightly.

Grate the cheese and set aside. Grate the cooked celeriac coarsely and set aside.

Put the eggs, the chopped dill, pepper and mustard into a large bowl and beat with a balloon whisk. Stir in the grated cheese, celeriac and leeks. Mix well.

Heat the non-stick omelette pan over a moderate heat and return the mixture to the pan, spreading it out and smoothing the top. Immediately reduce the heat to the lowest setting and cook for about 10 minutes.

Meanwhile, heat a grill/broiler, positioning the shelf 15 cm/6 in from the heat.

After the 10 minutes of cooking time on the top of the stove, the frittata mixture should be firming up around the edges. Place the pan under the grill and grill for another 8–10 minutes or until the mixture is firm all the way through and the top is golden. Slide or invert on to a serving plate.

SERVES 4 as a main meal
SERVES 8 in a selection of dishes

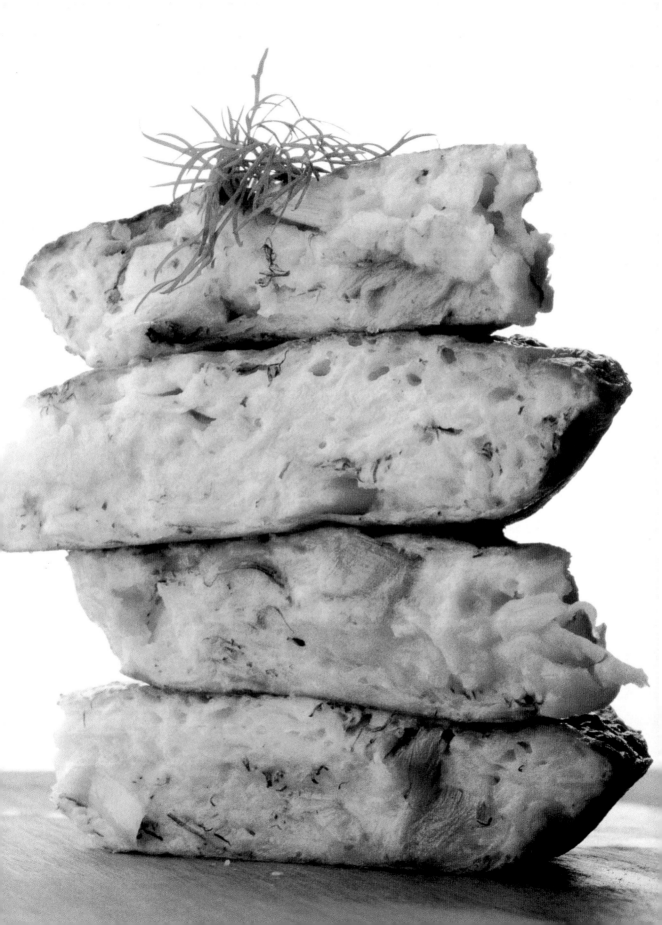

GRATED POTATO, PEA AND SPRING ONION FRITTERS

This makes a good lunch or light supper dish, served with the Spicy Tomato Sauce on page 103, or Roasted Plum Tomatoes (see page 42) and a Green Salad (see page 47).

	METRIC	IMPERIAL	CUPS
1 large potato, peeled and coarsely grated	300 g	10 ½ oz	2 cups
finely sliced spring onion/scallions, including the green tops (roughly 2 onions)		4 tbsp	
2 eggs, separated			
cornflour/cornstarch		½ tbsp	
lots of black pepper			
freshly grated nutmeg		1 tsp	
2 cloves garlic, crushed			
cooked peas		3 tbsp	
1 chilli pepper, seeded (see page 46), and finely chopped (optional)			
sunflower oil for frying			

Peel and grate the potato, then put into a colander to allow the juices to drain away.

In a large bowl, put the onion, egg yolks, cornflour, black pepper, nutmeg, garlic, peas and chilli if used. Mix well. Pat the potato with kitchen towel to dry it as much as possible, then put into the egg mixture and mix well using a fork.

Beat the egg whites to soft peaks. With a large metal spoon fold 1 spoonful into the potato mixture to soften it, then fold in the remaining egg whites very carefully.

Heat a small amount of sunflower oil in a frying pan/skillet over a moderate heat. The oil needs to be hot enough to cook the mixture quickly, otherwise it will absorb the oil.

Spoon a tablespoon of mixture into the oil and flatten gently with the spoon. The fritters should be thin to ensure that the potatoes are cooked in the centre. Once the edges of the fritter are nicely browned, gently turn over and fry the other side. Cook the remaining potatoes in batches, draining them well on kitchen paper and keeping them on a warm plate until all are cooked. Serve immediately.

MAKES 6 LARGE FRITTERS

Gerry West, who works with us at Buxton Foods, previously managed an alfalfa factory. She knows everything there is to know about sprouting beans, peas and seeds, and we thought it would be a good idea to include her comments.

PULSES

Sprouted pulses/legumes are not just good for you (containing vitamins B1, B2, C and iron), they are delicious too. You can choose from aduki/adzuki beans, mung beans, soya beans, chick-peas/garbanzo beans or Puy lentils (and large green lentils). Grow them individually or together to make a tasty, nourishing mixture to add to salads and sandwiches, or use in a stuffing for chicken, fish or marrow.

Before soaking your chosen pulses, pick over and discard any that are blemished or broken. Remove stones and grit, then place the pulses in a sieve and wash thoroughly. Soak them overnight in a jar or bowl, then rinse and drain morning and night for 2–3 days until the sprouts appear. For such an effortless task, the results are extremely rewarding.

ALFALFA SEEDS

Most of us are accustomed to Chinese style beansprouts – opaque, watery shoots used for their crunchy texture and bulk in stir-fries and salads – but not everyone has tried alfalfa sprouts.

Alfalfa sprouts are different. They have a nutty, peppery taste with plenty of texture and juiciness. Physically, they resemble tiny, curly cress-like shoots which are harvested just at the point when the two cotyledons (first leaves) appear and start to go green. They grow directly from seed, with just the help of water and light, and the whole process takes only a matter of days. Mixed with radish or fenugreek seeds, they take on an aromatic spicy pungency which adds something special to salads, sandwiches and starters.

Alfalfa is rich in vitamins C, D, E and K plus iron and phosphorus. Radish contains A, B, C, iron and phosphorus, and fenugreek A, C and iron. Sprouter kits are widely available at good health-food shops, and growing your own is so easy and satisfying.

STEAMED TOFU AND SPICED SPROUTED BEANS

This dish has a 'clean' satisfying taste and looks very pretty. More information about sprouting beans can be found on the previous page.

	METRIC	IMPERIAL	CUPS
tofu (buy 4 x 150g/5½ oz blocks, one per person)	600 g	1 lb 5 oz	
8 spring onions/scallions			
mixed sprouted beans (including chick-peas/garbanzo beans, green peas, red beans, mung beans, sunflower seeds etc.)	250 g	8 ½ oz	2 ¼ cups
2 cloves garlic, cut into very fine slices			
olive oil		4 tbsp	
sunflower oil		4 tbsp	
cayenne pepper		¼ tsp	
tomato purée/paste, or sun-dried tomato purée/paste		4 tbsp	
water		2 tbsp	
lemon juice		½ tbsp	
black pepper			
FOR THE GARNISH:			
a few sprigs of lamb's lettuce/corn salad or other greens (watercress, frisée etc.)			

Put the tofu on a chopping board and, holding firmly down with the palm of your hand, cut in half horizontally with a sharp knife. Put the tofu slices into a stainless-steel steamer and steam for a couple of minutes.

Stir-fry all the other ingredients with the exception of the tomato purée, water and lemon juice for a few minutes until heated through. Then add the tomato purée, water and lemon juice and black pepper to taste.

To serve, arrange a slice of tofu on each plate, cover with the bean mixture and then put another slice of tofu on top. Spoon some more of the bean mixture around the plate and top with the lamb's lettuce or garnish of your choice.

SERVES 4

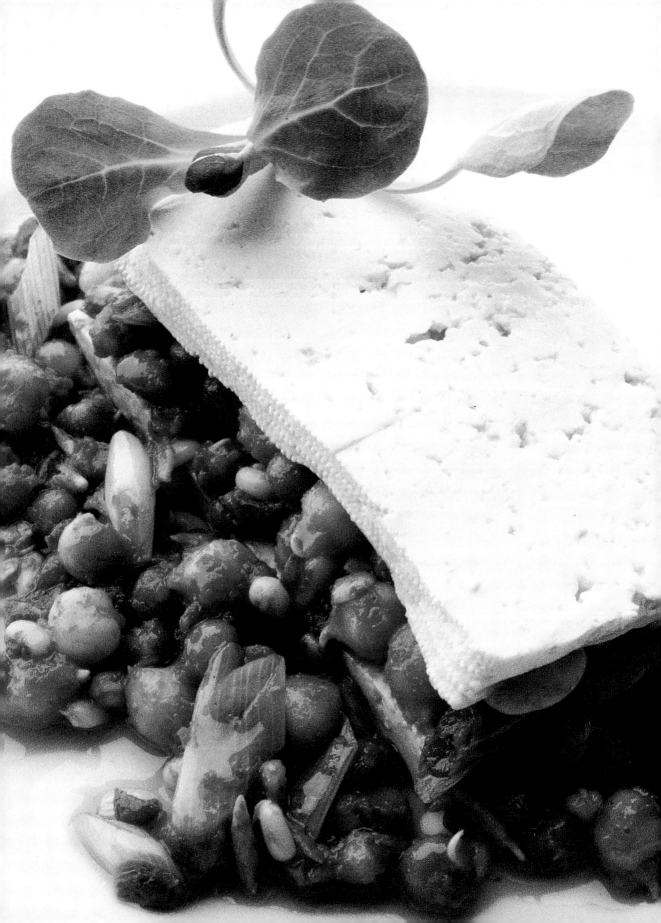

LIZ'S LUNCH TORTILLA

I often prepare this dish at night so that I can take it cold the following day for my packed lunch at the office.

	METRIC	IMPERIAL	CUPS
olive oil		2-3 tbsp	
1 celery stalk, chopped			
fresh ginger root, peeled and finely chopped		1 tsp	
1 medium or ½ large leek, chopped			
5 green cardamom pods, crushed			
turmeric		½ tsp	
cooked puy lentils	80 g	2½ oz	¾ cup
watercress, coarsely chopped	30 g	1 oz 3 tablespoons	
2 large eggs, beaten			
plenty of freshly ground black pepper			

Preheat the oven to 180°C/350°F/Gas 4.

Heat oil in a frying pan. Add the celery, ginger and leek and sauté over medium heat for 5 minutes. Add the cardamom and turmeric and fry for a couple of minutes. The vegetables should be softening but still firm.

Put the cooked lentils, chopped watercress and cooked leek mixture into a mixing bowl, scraping the spices and oil out of the pan with a spatula. Mix in the beaten eggs and black pepper.

Lightly oil an 18 cm/7 in non-stick baking tin. Pour in the mixture and bake for 20 minutes or until firm to the touch in the centre.

Cool and turn out. Cut into wedges to serve.

SERVES 2

AUBERGINES AND RED ONION WITH TWO GOAT'S CHEESES

This is a favourite with our vegetarian and non-vegetarian friends alike. It can mostly be prepared in advance and is a good party standby.

	METRIC	IMPERIAL	CUPS
4 large aubergines/eggplants			
olive oil for cooking			
1 large red onion, roughly sliced			
black pepper			
dried thyme		1 tbsp	
goat's cream cheese, coarsely grated	300 g	10½ oz	2 cups
goat's Cheddar cheese, coarsely grated	115 g	4 oz	1 cup

Cut the aubergines in half lengthways. Fry in olive oil, cut side down first. Turn when aubergines are golden and softening, then cook on the skin side until cooked through. Drain on kitchen paper. Using the same pan, fry the roughly sliced onion in the oil, but leave it quite firm and crunchy. Place the aubergines on a baking tray, cut side up. Sprinkle liberally with pepper, dried thyme and onions.* Cut the cream cheese into chunks and dot over the aubergines then cover completely with the grated Cheddar. Grill/broil until golden brown.

* May be prepared to this point a day in advance and refrigerated.

SERVES 4

WILD MUSHROOMS AND AUTUMN VEGETABLES WITH POTATO CAKES

This is a very rich dish and is ideal for festive occasions. We have suggested using wild mushrooms, but button or chestnut mushrooms will do just as well. The secret is to prepare all the vegetables ahead of time and cook them just before serving. The vegetables should be only just cooked and still have a certain 'bite'; they will go mushy if they are overcooked.

	METRIC	IMPERIAL	CUPS
FOR THE AUTUMN VEGETABLES:			
carrots	170 g	6 oz	
Jerusalem artichokes	275 g	9 oz	
olive oil		2 tbsp	
balsamic vinegar		½ tbsp	
FOR THE POTATO CAKES:			
main-crop potatoes	450 g	1 lb	
1 egg, beaten			
freshly grated nutmeg		⅛ tsp	
plenty of black pepper to taste			
fine oatmeal to dust	30 g	1 oz	¼ cup
sunflower oil for frying			
FOR THE MUSHROOMS:			
shiitake mushrooms, sliced	90 g	3 oz	1½ cup
field mushrooms, quartered	90 g	3 oz	1½ cup
wild mushrooms of your choice, left whole	90 g	3 oz	
olive oil	175 ml	6 fl oz	¾ cup
spring onions/scallions cut into 2.5 cm/1 in pieces	115 g	4 oz	⅔ cup
good pinch cayenne pepper			
lemon juice		1½ tbsp	
freshly ground black pepper to taste			
2 cloves garlic, finely sliced			
tomato purée/paste		1½ tbsp	
a big handful flat parsley with stalks, chopped			

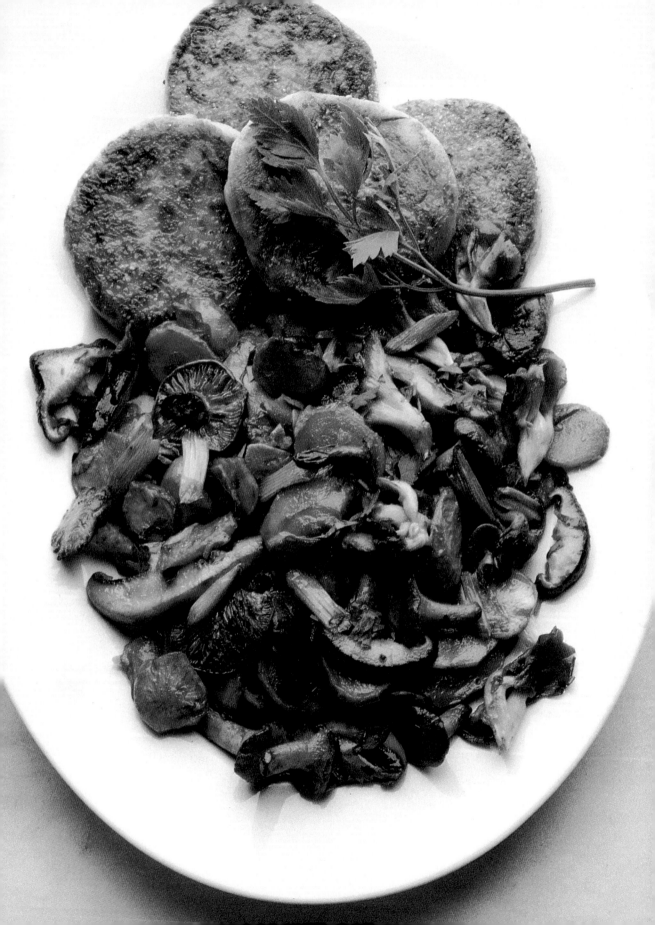

WILD MUSHROOMS AND AUTUMN VEGETABLES WITH POTATO CAKES continued

Preheat the oven to its highest setting. Peel and slice the vegetables. Slice the carrots diagonally to half the thickness of the Jerusalem artichokes. I would suggest that the carrots be sliced 3mm/$\frac{1}{8}$ in thick and the artichokes 6mm/$\frac{1}{4}$ in thick. Put the slices into a mixing bowl and pour over the oil and vinegar. Toss so that the vegetables are coated then spread out in a roasting tray so that there is only one layer of vegetables. Roast for 20 minutes. When cooked the vegetables should not be soft, but still have a bit of bite.

Meanwhile prepare the potatoes. Boil them until they are soft. Drain, peel and mash off the heat. Stir in the beaten egg and the seasoning. Divide the mixture into 4 portions. With your hands, form flat patties. Put the oatmeal on to a plate and carefully coat the flat surfaces of the potato cakes.

While the potatoes are boiling and the carrots and artichokes are roasting, prepare the mushroom ingredients.

When the carrots and artichokes are ready and the potato cakes have been formed, get 2 frying pans/skillets and assemble the dish. This will only take about 5 minutes.

In one frying pan heat put just enough sunflower oil to coat the bottom of the pan and fry the potato cakes in the medium hot oil, turning when golden and crispy.

In the other frying pan heat the olive oil for the mushrooms. Put in the spring onions and stir-fry for 1 minute. Add the cayenne pepper, the lemon juice, black pepper and garlic and cook, stirring, for another minute. Add the tomato purée and stir to mix well. Add the mushrooms, cooked carrots and artichokes and fry, turning the ingredients over constantly for a couple of minutes or until cooked through but still firm. Stir in the roughly chopped parsley, adjust seasoning to taste and serve immediately with the hot potato cakes.

SERVES 4

POTATO BAKE

This makes a hearty meal served with steamed spinach or a green salad.

	METRIC	IMPERIAL	CUPS
8 large waxy potatoes, roughly cut into pieces			
olive oil		3 tbsp	
8 tomatoes, roughly chopped			
1 clove garlic, crushed			
1 hot small red chilli, seeded and chopped (see page 46)			
½ stick lemongrass, finely sliced			
black pepper and lemon juice to taste			
1 bunch fresh coriander/cilantro, chopped			
hard cheese of your choice, grated	115 g	4 oz	1 cup

Preheat the oven to 190ºC/375ºF/Gas 5.Put the olive oil into a baking dish large enough for the potatoes to fit into it in one layer. Sprinkle over the tomatoes and bake until tender, about 1 hour. Half way through the cooking time add the garlic, chilli, lemongrass, pepper and lemon juice. Make sure that the potatoes are not sticking to the dish; turn the mixture over with a spatula. When the potatoes are tender, sprinkle with the coriander and cheese, and brown under the preheated grill/broiler.

SERVES 4

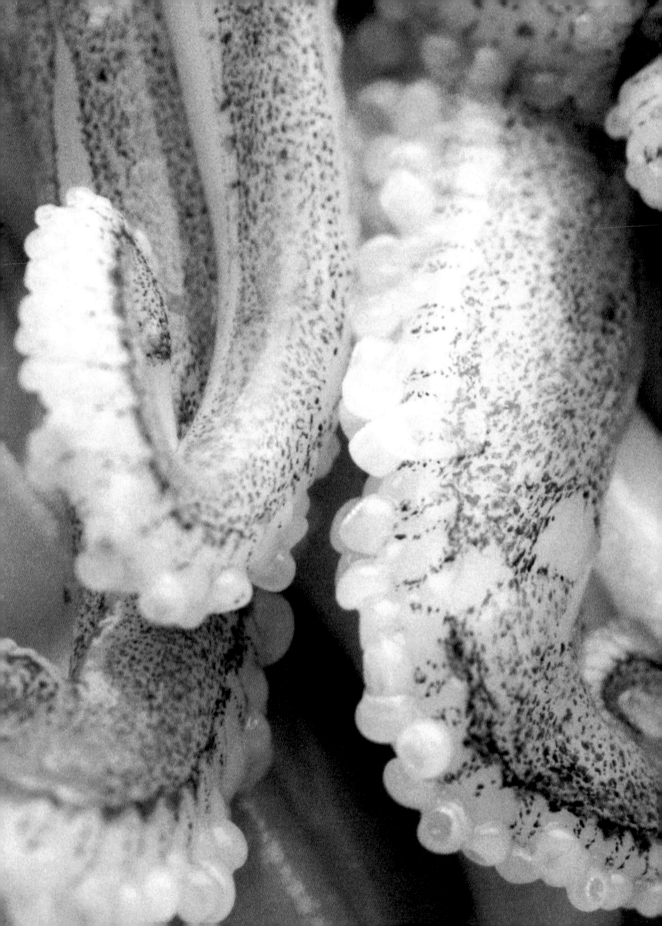

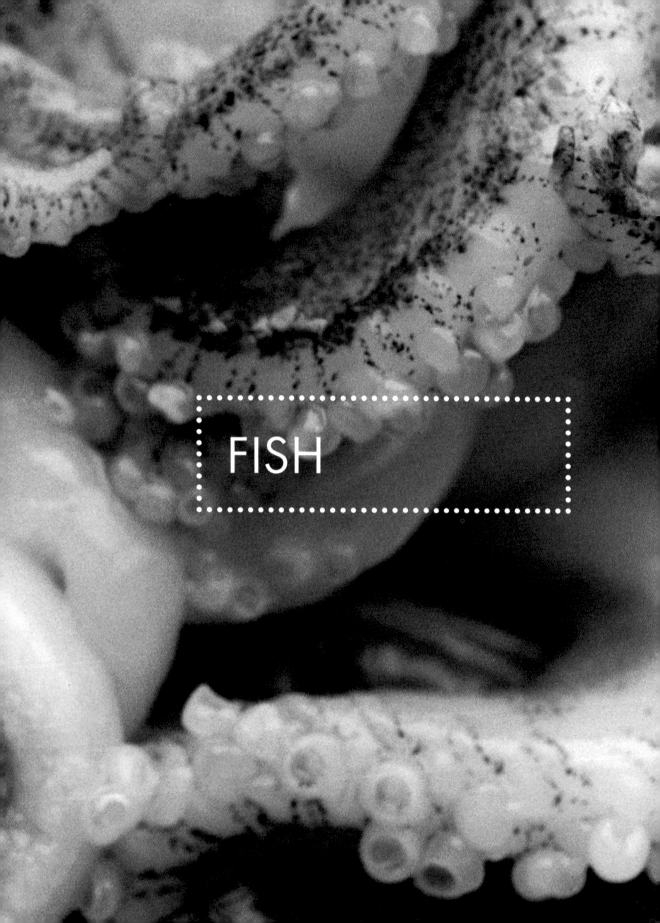

FISH

ROASTED SALMON WITH SULTANAS AND JAPANESE GINGER

This is my sister Anne's recipe. It is quick to make and is extremely pretty. Definitely festive enough for any party gathering.

	METRIC	IMPERIAL	CUPS
4 fillets of salmon	115 g each	4 oz each	
sultanas/golden raisins		2 tbsp	
olive oil		½ tsp	
1–2 lemons			
black pepper			
fresh coriander/cilantro leaves		2 tbsp	
Japanese pickled ginger (available from some supermarkets and speciality stores)		2 tbsp	

Put the sultanas in a small bowl and pour over some boiling water. Leave to soak until plump – about 15–20 minutes.

Preheat the oven to its hottest setting. Thoroughly oil a baking tray and place into the oven.

Squeeze the lemon juice over the fish on all sides and grind over black pepper to taste.

Put the drained sultanas, coriander and ginger into a small bowl and, using kitchen scissors, roughly chop. Divide this mixture and arrange on the top of each salmon fillet. Place on the hot baking tray and bake for about 15 minutes or until the fish is opaque, depending on the thickness of the fillets.

SERVES 4

SQUID AND POTATO STEW

Squid may not be top of everybody's shopping list but this has been a family favourite for years. Served hot, it is a wonderfully satisfying dish in winter and, served cold with additional lemon juice and olive oil, it makes an unusual summer salad. The flavours improve if it is prepared a day in advance. This is a hearty dish and should resemble a stew with the potatoes cooked through but not mushy. Ask your fishmonger to clean the squid thoroughly. If you do not like the look or texture of the tentacles, ask that he only supplies you with the body part of the squid.

	METRIC	IMPERIAL	CUPS
squid, cleaned and cut into 1 cm/½ in slices	450 g	1 lb	
olive oil	125 ml	4 fl oz	½ cup
3 cloves garlic, crushed			
small waxy potatoes, scrubbed and cut in half	450 g	1 lb	
can tomatoes	1 x 250 g	1 x 8½ oz	
tomato purée/paste		1 tsp	
white wine vinegar	60 ml	2 fl oz	¼ cup
water	125 ml	4 fl oz	½ cup
juice of at least 1 lemon and more to taste if required			
seasonings to taste			
large bunch fresh thyme			

Heat the oil in a sauté dish that has a lid and toss the squid and garlic in the hot oil for a few minutes or until the squid turns opaque. Off the heat add all the other ingredients and then cover and cook over a low heat until the potatoes are cooked but still firm, stirring from time to time. Depending upon the amount of liquid in the tomatoes and the amount of liquid absorbed by the potatoes, it may be necessary to add some more water during the cooking. Adjust seasoning before eating, adding more oil, lemon juice and pepper to taste.

SERVES 4

MUSSEL, PARSNIP, FENNEL AND LEEK RAGOUT

	METRIC	IMPERIAL	CUPS
mussels, in their shells	900 g	2 lb	
2 large parsnips			
2 large leeks			
1 fennel bulb			
olive oil	125 ml	4 fl oz	½ cup
tomato purée/paste		2 tbsp	
paprika		¼ tsp	
turmeric		¼ tsp	
2 pinches cayenne pepper			
lemon juice		1 tbsp	
Worcestershire sauce		1 tbsp	
water	250 ml	8 fl oz	1 cup
cornflour/cornstarch		2 tsp	
sheep's yogurt	250 ml	8 fl oz	1 cup

Rinse the mussels in plenty of cold running water. Leave to stand for an hour in cold water, changing the water from time to time. Remove the fibrous 'beard' and discard any mussels that are open or have broken shells. Rinse again under cold running water and stand in cold water until ready for use.

Peel the parsnips and top and tail them. Slice diagonally in 6mm/¼ in slices. Trim the leeks, discarding any tough outer leaves. Wash thoroughly then slice in 2.5 cm/1 in long sections. Cut the fennel in half lengthways and slice horizontally in 1 cm/½ in pieces.

Heat the oil in the bottom saucepan half of a steamer, and cook the vegetables in it for 2 minutes. Add the tomato purée and spices and stir in well. Add the lemon juice, Worcestershire sauce and water. Place the mussels in the steamer above the vegetables, cover and steam for about 5 minutes or until the shells open. The juice will drop into the vegetable mixture. Remove from the heat. Quickly take the mussels out of the shells and put them into the vegetables, leaving in the steamer about 6 mussels per person in their shells for decoration. Discard any mussels that have not opened. Mix the cornflour into the yogurt in a small bowl using a balloon whisk, then whisk into the soup. Return the mixture to the heat and bring gently to the boil, stirring for a couple of minutes. The liquid will thicken slightly. Serve immediately in individual bowls, topped with the remaining steamed mussels.

SERVES 4

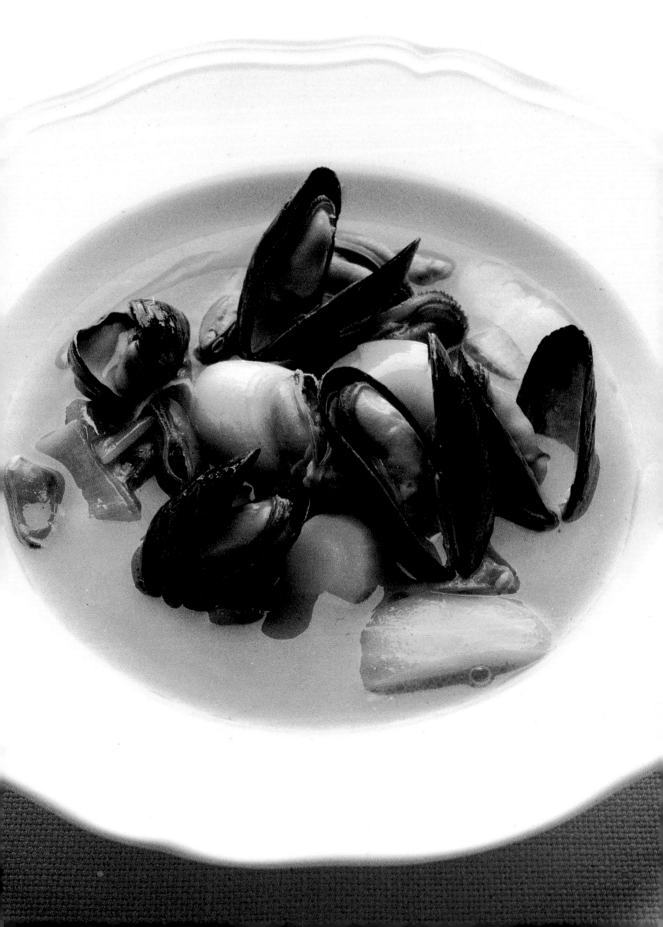

MONKFISH AND STUFFED MUSHROOMS

Most weekends, Lucy and I visit our favourite fishmonger. We have more time then and can stop to have a good chat. There is nothing Simon does not know about the fish he sells: where they were caught, which are the freshest and the best ways to prepare them. Simon only sells wild or organically farmed fish.

The stuffed mushrooms in this recipe can be used as part of a vegetarian meal or on their own as a starter.

	METRIC	IMPERIAL	CUPS
monkfish, skinned, boned and cut into 2.5 cm/1 in chunks	350 g	12 oz	
juice of ½ lemon			
FOR THE STUFFED MUSHROOMS:			
8 large flat field mushrooms			
olive oil			
1 red onion, chopped			
1 yellow bell pepper, seeded and chopped			
1 small mild chilli, seeded and finely chopped, (see page 46)			
1 clove garlic, very finely chopped/minced			
cooked organic brown rice	800 g	1¾ lb	4 cups
black pepper to taste			
finely grated pecorino cheese		4 tbsp	
FOR THE THICK BECHAMEL SAUCE (see page 153):			
margarine	45 g	1½ oz	3 tbsp
all-purpose wheat-free flour		3 tbsp	
sheep's or goat's milk	125 ml	4 fl oz	½ cup
Dijon mustard		½ tsp	
nutmeg to taste			

Make the béchamel sauce first as described on page 153. Then preheat the oven to 200°C/400°F/ Gas 6.

Carefully remove the stalks from the mushrooms and chop roughly. Put 1 tbsp olive oil in a non-stick pan with the chopped onion, yellow pepper and mushroom stalks. Cook until the vegetables start to become tender. Add the finely chopped chilli pepper and garlic and cook for 1 minute. Add the cooked rice and béchamel to the contents of the pan. Place the mushroom caps, gill side up, on a greased baking tray. Stuff with the mixture, sprinkle with grated cheese and drizzle with olive oil. Bake for 20 minutes.

When ready to serve, cook the monkfish in a preheated non-stick frying pan/skillet, dry and without oil, until the fish has turned opaque. Sprinkle with lemon juice and serve with the stuffed mushrooms and green vegetables or salad.

SERVES 4

CHAR-GRILLED TUNA STEAKS WITH MINT SALSA SAUCE

Cooking the tuna creates a lot of smoke, so shut the kitchen door and open all the windows, turn on the extractor fan – or cook outside!

	METRIC	IMPERIAL	CUPS
6 very fresh tuna steaks, cut 1 cm/½ in thick			
a little olive oil			
freshly ground black pepper			
FOR THE MINT SALSA:			
fresh mint leaves	30 g	1 oz	½ cup
3 jalapeño chillies, whole with their seeds, but with stalks removed			
sunflower oil		3 tbsp	
olive oil		2 tbsp	
lemon juice		4 tbsp	
warm water		1 tbsp	

Put a grill pan over a high heat to get really hot while you prepare the salsa sauce.

Put all the salsa ingredients into a food processor and blend.

To cook the tuna, brush one side of the tuna steaks with a little olive oil and grind over plenty of black pepper. When the grill pan is very hot, place the tuna steaks on it, oiled side down. When the fish starts to go opaque around the edges, brush the top side with oil and sprinkle with black pepper as before, turn and cook for a further 1–2 minutes depending on the thickness of the steaks, and depending on your preference for well cooked or 'pink' tuna.

Pour a generous helping of the mint salsa over a quarter of the tuna steak and around it on the plate.

SERVES 6

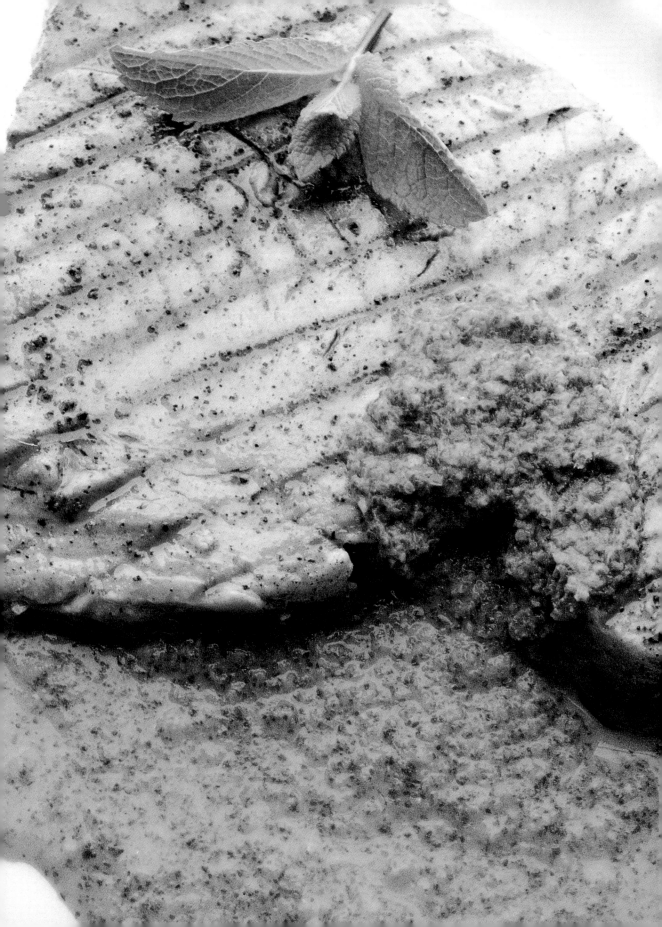

FISH PIE

If at all possible buy the prawns in the shell – the texture and colour are so much better than the frozen peeled variety. Almost any fresh herbs can be used and any firm fleshed fish.

	METRIC	IMPERIAL	CUPS
firm white fish	675g	1 ½ lb	2 cups
peeled prawns/shrimp	55 g	2 oz	1 cup
4 hard-boiled eggs, chopped in eighths			
mashed potato	400–600 g	14–20 oz	2–3 cups
grated goat's Cheddar cheese	55 g	2 oz	½ cup
FOR THE SAUCE:			
sunflower oil		3 tbsp	
all-purpose wheat-free flour		3 tbsp	
Dijon mustard		1 tsp	
sweet paprika powder		½ tsp	
chopped mixed fresh herbs (chives, dill and tarragon)	55 g	2 oz	1 cup
sheep or goat's milk	600 ml	1 pt	2 ½ cups
grated goat's Cheddar cheese	55 g	2 oz	½ cup
black pepper			

Preheat the oven to 240°C/475°F/Gas 9. Make the sauce first. Put the oil in a pan, then add the flour off the heat and cook, stirring, for 2 minutes. Add the mustard, paprika and herbs and stir in the milk. Return to the heat and stir until boiling. The mixture should be the consistency of thick cream, so add more milk if necessary. Remove from the heat, and stir in the grated cheese and some black pepper.

To cook the fish, put it in a pan, just covered with water, bring to the boil and turn the heat off immediately. Allow to stand in the hot water until the flesh turns opaque. Drain and flake into large pieces, removing any bones.

In an ovenproof dish, place the ingredients in layers, first the flaked white fish, then the prawns, then the chopped eggs. Pour over the sauce, shaking the dish slightly to ensure that it runs down through the ingredients. The top layer should be just covered by the sauce. Using a spatula, cover with the mashed potatoes and then sprinkle with the cheese. Bake in the hot oven for 15 minutes until bubbling and heated through, and finish under the grill/broiler to get a golden crust.

SERVES 4

SPICY SEAFOOD STIR-FRY

This is a recipe that includes a selection of fish and shellfish chosen for their variety of colour, shape and texture.

	METRIC	IMPERIAL	CUPS
4 scallops with their corals			
1 large squid, cleaned			
8 large raw tiger prawns (or jumbo shrimp)			
olive oil		1 tbsp	
1 clove garlic, chopped			
1 small red chilli, chopped and seeded (see page 46)			
2.5 cm/1 in fresh ginger root, peeled and chopped			
1 stick lemongrass, chopped			
zest and juice of 1 lime			
rice wine (optional)		2 tbsp	
chopped fresh coriander/cilantro			

Separate the corals and discard the white gristly bit from the scallops. Cut the scallops in half horizontally. Cut the squid into strips. Cut the tentacles into bite-sized pieces. Peel the prawns, remove the black vein and cut in half lengthways.

In a heavy non-stick pan, heat the oil and stir-fry the garlic, chilli, ginger and lemongrass for a few minutes. Add the fish and toss until it turns opaque. Add the lime zest, juice and rice wine and boil rapidly for 1 minute. Add fresh coriander.

Serve with boiled rice or rice noodles.

SKATE WITH CAPER BERRIES AND BLACK OLIVES

This recipe combines two of Terence Stamp's favourite foods, skate and caper berries. It is a simple variation of the French classic, Raie au Beurre Noire.

	METRIC	IMPERIAL	CUPS
4 pieces of skate wing			
all-purpose wheat-free flour		4 tbsp	
black pepper			
olive oil	80 ml	2 ¾ fl oz	⅓ cup
sunflower oil	80 ml	2 ¾ fl oz	⅓ cup
juice of 1 lemon			
FOR THE GARNISH:			
zest of 2 lemons			
20 caper berries (the stalks are edible)			
12 stoned/pitted black olives, roughly chopped			
4 sprigs flat parsley			

Dust the fish in the flour mixed with the pepper. Fry the fish in the heated oils for 2–3 minutes on either side. Drain and set aside in a hot serving dish.

Tilt the frying pan/skillet and spoon off 4 tbsp of the cooking oil into a small saucepan, being careful to leave the sediment behind. Add the lemon juice to the oil and spoon this mixture over the fish. Divide the garnish ingredients evenly – lemon zest, caper berries, olives and parsley – and arrange over the fish. Serve immediately.

Very good served with Roasted Plum Tomatoes (see page 42) and plain boiled waxy potatoes.

SERVES 4

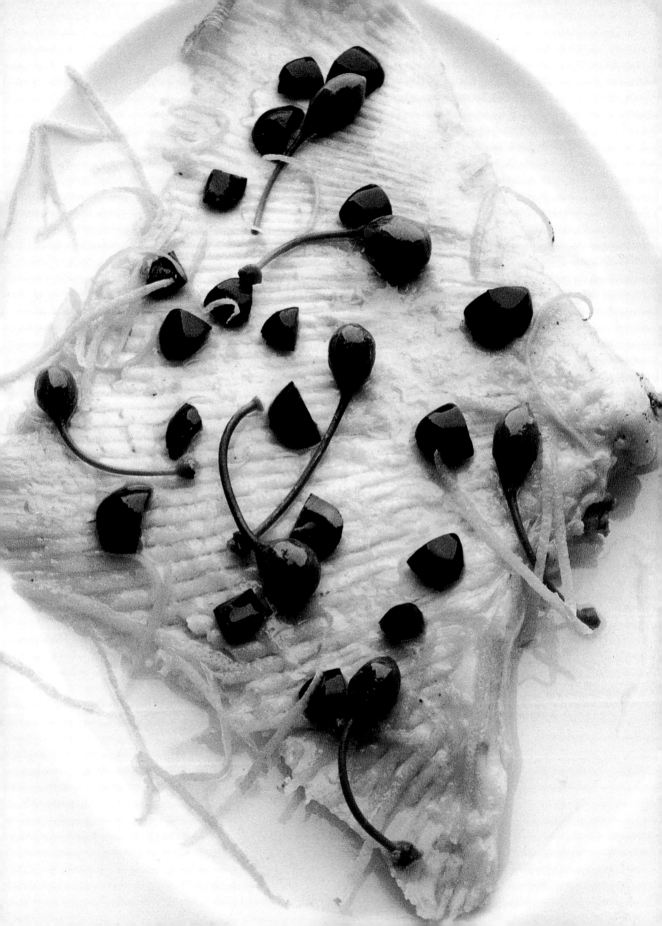

CRAB CAKES

Every summer we go on a crabbing expedition. The time and tide need to be just right. Early morning is best, at low tide when the crabs are trapped in the shallow water behind a sand bar. It is surprisingly difficult. The crabs are very well camouflaged and can run much faster than a small child wielding a net. Simple steamed crabs with fresh corn is best, but if we have had a good catch we also make these crab cakes.

	METRIC	IMPERIAL	CUPS
prepared white crab meat (fresh, canned or frozen)	450 g	1 lb	4 cups
3 medium potatoes, boiled, peeled and mashed			
1 clove garlic, chopped			
chilli flakes or fresh green chilli, seeded and chopped (see page 46)		½ tsp	
1 spring onion/scallion, sliced (white and green parts)			
sunflower oil			
Dijon mustard		1 tsp	
juice of ½ lemon			
black pepper			
1 egg, beaten			
a little oatmeal for dusting			

Fry the garlic, chilli and onion in 2 tbsp oil for a few minutes but do not allow to colour.

Put the crab and mashed potatoes into a mixing bowl. Add the garlic, oil mixture, mustard, lemon juice and black pepper and stir. Bind with the beaten egg. Form into patties and coat with oatmeal. Refrigerate for at least 15 minutes, then fry in shallow sunflower oil until golden brown on both sides.

SERVES 4

SEAFOOD SPAGHETTI

Organic wheat-free spaghetti has the true 'bite' of Italian pasta and so is ideal to feed to your friends and family who do not have a wheat intolerance – they won't know the difference!

	METRIC	IMPERIAL	CUPS
12 small clams in their shells, cleaned			
squid, cleaned and sliced into rings	100 g	3½ oz	
olive oil	100 ml	3½ fl oz	½ cup
garlic, finely chopped		1 tbsp	
chilli flakes		½ tsp (or to taste)	
flat parsley, chopped	15 g	½ oz	⅓ cup
cooked and peeled prawns/shrimp	100 g	3½ oz	1¾ cups
fresh organic wheat-free spaghetti	250 g	8½ oz	
2 large prawns/shrimp, to garnish			
a few sprigs of parsley, to garnish			

Put 1 cm/½ in water in the bottom of a double boiler and add the clams. Place the squid in the top steamer. Place the double boiler over a high heat for a couple of minutes, shaking the pan from time to time. The clams are cooked once the shells have opened and the squid is cooked when it turns white. Remove from the heat.

Heat the oil in a large sauté pan. Add the garlic and cook for 2 minutes, without browning. Add the chilli flakes and parsley and cook for a further minute. Add the shrimp, squid and clams and stir to coat in flavoured oil.

Meanwhile, cook the spaghetti according to the instructions on the pack. Drain the spaghetti, reheat the fish mixture (if necessary) and add the spaghetti. Mix well and divide onto two plates, topping each with a large prawn and parsley sprigs.

SERVES 2

SCALLOPS WITH GARLIC POTATOES, WATERCRESS AND RED ONION

This is the simplest, quickest dish to make. As with all seafood, it is essential to use really fresh scallops for the best results.

	METRIC	IMPERIAL	CUPS
scallops with their coral	450 g	1 lb	
small waxy potatoes, scrubbed	450 g	1 lb	
olive oil	125 ml	4 fl oz	½ cup
2 cloves garlic, crushed			
black pepper			
chilli flakes (optional)		¼ tsp	
lemon juice			
watercress	75 g	2 ½ oz	
4–5 slices red onion, rings separated			

Remove any tough white membrane from the scallops and cut in half horizontally. If there is coral, try and keep this attached to one half of the scallops as this will reduce their shrinkage.

Boil the potatoes until only just cooked through (about 10–15 minutes). They should be firm.

The next stage will only take a couple of minutes so do this just before sitting down to eat. Cut the potatoes in half and put in a sauté pan with the oil, garlic, black pepper and chilli (if used) and toss. Reheat over a medium heat, making sure that the garlic does not colour.

Meanwhile, brush a non-stick frying pan/skillet with a little oil, removing any excess with kitchen paper, and heat the pan. When it is hot, dry-fry the scallops and sear on both sides until just cooked through. This will only take 1–2 minutes, depending upon the thickness of the sliced scallops. Turn them over when the edges start to go white and cook on the other side. The scallops will caramelize and char slightly. Squeeze a little lemon juice over each piece, with black pepper to taste.

Toss the watercress and onion into the hot potato mixture, off the heat. They should not cook or wilt, but be well coated with the garlic oil. Season to taste, top with the scallops and serve immediately.

SERVES 4 as a main dish

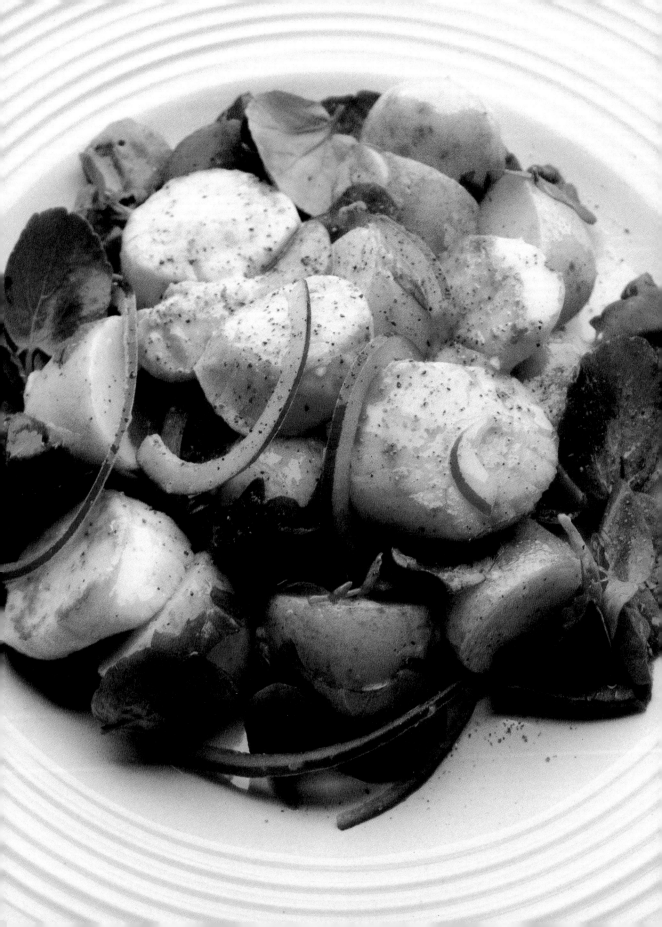

TUNA AND CHICK-PEA SALAD

This is ideal for unexpected guests because most of the ingredients come from the store-cupboard. Prawns can be used instead of the tuna.

	METRIC	IMPERIAL	CUPS
can chick-peas/garbanzo beans, well rinsed	1 x 400 g	1 x 14 oz	
cooked peas, fresh or frozen	425 g	15 oz	2 3/4 cups
5 tomatoes, roughly chopped into bite-sized pieces			
cooked fresh tuna, or canned	400 g	14 oz	
2 tbsp each of coarsely chopped fresh basil, chives and parsley			
juice of 1/2 lemon			
black pepper to taste			
olive oil		2 tbsp	

Mix all the ingredients in bowl and serve at room temperature – or chill if preferred.

SERVES 4

COD WITH JALAPENO PEPPER AND DILL COATING

This is extremely simple to cook and prepare. Serve it with the colourful Corn, Tomato, Red Onion and Avocado Salad on page 44, with extra lime juice added. This will cool down and balance the fieriness of the chillies.

	METRIC	IMPERIAL	CUPS
2 jalapeño chilli peppers, whole including the seeds, but with stalk removed			
3 cloves garlic			
grated rind of 1 lemon			
juice of ½ lemon			
1 handful fresh dill	20 g	½ oz	¼ cup
1 handful fresh parsley leaves	20 g	½ oz	¼ cup
olive oil		1 tbsp	
4 cod fillets or other firm white fish			

In a liquidizer blend all the ingredients together – except for the fish! Place the fish fillets on an oiled baking tray, skin side down. Coat the top side of the fish with the herb mixture and allow to marinate for at least 1 hour.

Preheat the oven to its hottest temperature and place the fish in the centre of the oven for 6–10 minutes according to the thickness of the fish. The fish will turn opaque when it is cooked through.

SERVES 4

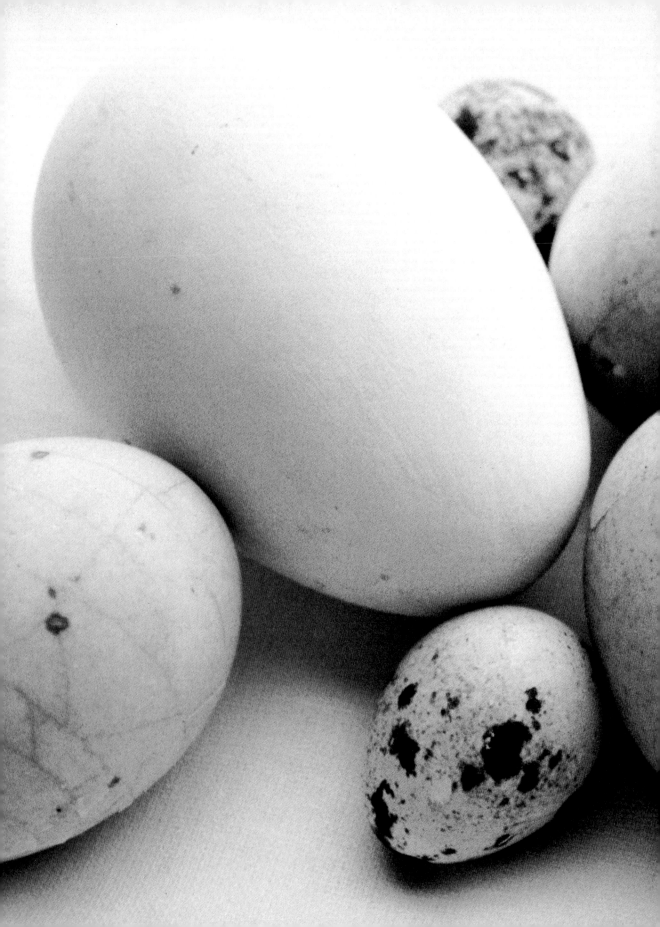

FOWL

CHICKEN NIÇOISE

This dish is delicious served hot with a simple saffron risotto, but is also very good cold with a rice salad. To serve it cold, simply arrange it on a shallow serving dish and sprinkle with roasted pine kernels.

	METRIC	IMPERIAL	CUPS
2 sweet onions, each cut into eighths through the base			
olive oil	60 ml	2 fl oz	¼ cup
1 green bell pepper, cut into chunks			
1 yellow bell pepper, cut into chunks			
1 red bell pepper, cut into chunks			
1 good pinch of chilli flakes			
chicken stock	250 ml	8 fl oz	1 cup
1 can chopped tomatoes	225 g	8 oz	1 cup
pitted/stoned black olives, sliced	100 g	3½ oz	¾ cup
½ large cooked chicken, cut off the bone into large pieces			
lemon juice and black pepper to taste			
fresh flat parsley, roughly chopped		1 tbsp	

In a large pan over a high heat, sauté the onions in oil for 5 minutes. Add the peppers and continue to cook until the vegetables are beginning to soften and are slightly charred. Add the chilli flakes and fry for 1 minute, stirring constantly.

Pour in the chicken stock, scraping up any residues from the bottom of the pan. Add the chopped tomatoes, olives and chicken, mixing thoroughly until all the ingredients are heated through.

Season to taste with lemon juice and black pepper, sprinkle over parsley and serve immediately.

SERVES 4

ROAST CHICKEN

This is the simplest way to roast a chicken and is the method that gives the best results. A 900 g/2 lb chicken will feed six people, for use in the recipe overleaf. Roast a larger bird and use leftover meat in a variety of ways. We have included several recipes for cold roast chicken and these can be found on pages 96, 98 and 106. Always save the bones for stock; see two methods for this on page 155. If possible use an organic bird, as the flavour and texture are so much better; and because the animal is healthy, the bones are much larger and make good stock for soup (see page 155). The liver is wonderful and can be used for pâté (see page 24) or pan-roasted and served with corn fritters (see page 28).

Preheat the oven to 220°C/425°F/Gas 7.

Rinse the bird thoroughly under cold running water, allowing the water to run through the body cavity. Put the bird in a roasting pan filled with water 2.5 cm/1 in deep. Arrange the giblets round the bird, excluding the liver and crop. Put in the hot oven for 20 minutes per 450 g/1 lb, depending upon the plumpness of the bird. Remove the bird from the oven and pierce the thickest area, usually the lower thigh, with a skewer. If the juices run out clear, the bird is cooked. If the juices are at all pink return to the oven for a further 10 minutes and test again.

The water in the pan has two functions it gives off a steam so the bird is being steamed and roasted at the same time. This keeps the meat juicy while allowing the skin to crisp. The second function is to provide you with a 'jus' which can be served with the carved meat.

Put the cooked bird on a warm carving platter and allow to 'rest' for at least 5 minutes before carving. It will retain its heat for much longer in fact, and this will give you time to make the gravy and assemble the other vegetables being served.

Put the roasting pan on the top of the stove and carefully scrape up all the sediments. Add a little boiling water or any water over which accompanying vegetables have been steamed. Turn on the heat, bring to the boil and season to taste.

Personally I prefer this simple 'jus' to a thickened gravy. If you would like a thickened gravy, add 1–2 tsp cornflour/cornstarch to the roasting pan juices when removed from the oven and before pouring in the extra liquid. Whisk in to incorporate and remove any lumps. Add the extra liquid, bring to the boil, boil for 2 minutes, season and serve.

SERVES 6

ROAST CHICKEN WITH OKRA PROVENÇAL

I am lucky to live close to an organic butcher. Mohamad is full of good recipe suggestions. Here is one of them using dried okra which is available from his shop, threaded like a necklace on a length of string. This is the only ingredient that we have included in this book that may be difficult to find unless you live near a shop that sells Middle Eastern produce. Fresh, canned or frozen okra may be substituted, reducing the overall cooking time accordingly, but do try and seek out the dried. It has none of the gelatinous character of the fresh vegetable, is small, holds its shape and tastes simply delicious.

	METRIC	IMPERIAL	CUPS
1 small roast chicken, jointed (see page 95) or cooked chicken pieces	900 g	2 lb	
1 strand of dried okra (makes up to about 285 g/10 oz after initial soaking)	90 g	3 oz	
olive oil	60 ml	2 fl oz	¼ cup
finely chopped garlic		1 heaped tbsp	
lemon juice		2½ tbsp	
plenty of freshly ground black pepper			
cans chopped tomatoes	2 x 400 g	2 x 14 oz	
water	60 ml	2 fl oz	¼ cup
fresh coriander/cilantro, coarsely chopped	25 g	1 oz	

Unthread the dried okra. Put into a bowl and cover with boiling water. Let stand for 1 hour. Drain.

Preheat the oven to 180°C/350°F/Gas 4.

Put the olive oil into a flameproof casserole dish that is large enough to hold the okra and the chicken. Sauté the chopped garlic and the drained okra for 2 minutes. Add the lemon juice, black pepper, tomatoes, water and 20 g/³⁄₄ oz of the chopped coriander, then return to the heat and boil rapidly for 2 minutes. Cover the casserole and cook in the oven for 30 minutes. Add the cooked chicken pieces, submerging them in the tomato and okra mixture and continue to cook in the oven for another 30 minutes.

Sprinkle over the remaining coriander, and serve with boiled potatoes pushed through a potato ricer or rice.

SERVES 6

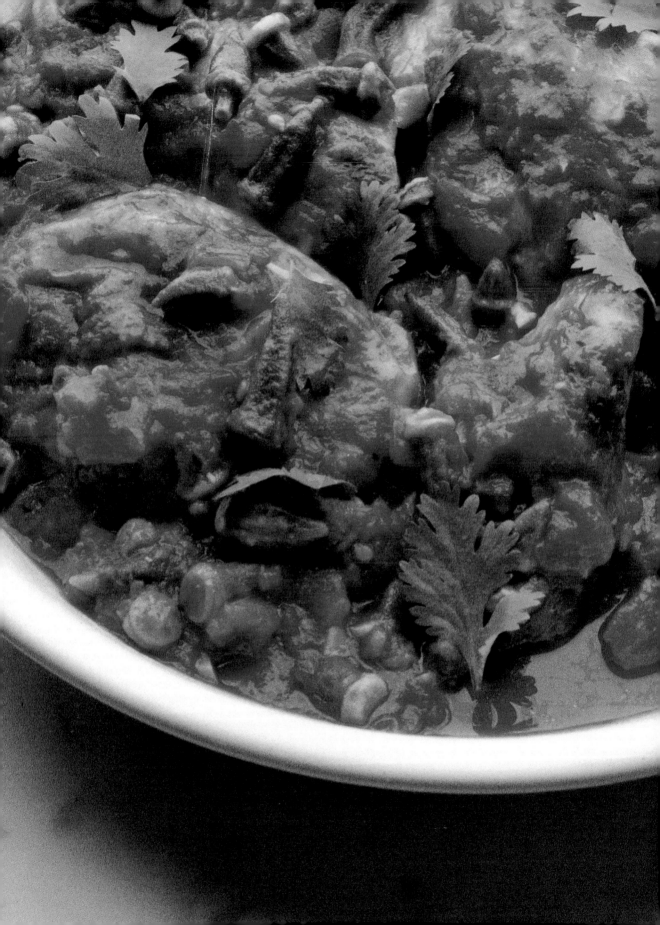

CHICKEN WITH CREAMED COCONUT AND AROMATIC SPICES

This is a good way to revive leftover cooked chicken. Chillies vary greatly in strength. I use the pale green Mexican chillies for this dish as they are quite mild. If you find the sauce to be too hot, add more yogurt to cool it down.

	METRIC	IMPERIAL	CUPS
chicken, cut into chunks (this can be cold leftover chicken or fresh)	225 g	8 oz	
1 medium onion, roughly chopped			
vegetable oil		3 tbsp	
1 green bell pepper, cut into 2.5 cm/1 in squares			
2 cloves garlic, finely chopped			
2.5 cm/1 in fresh ginger root, peeled and finely chopped			
1 fresh chilli, finely chopped (see page 46)			
turmeric		$1/2$ tsp	
paprika		$1/2$ tsp	
ground cinnamon		$1/4$ tsp	
creamed coconut	150 ml	$1/4$ pt	$2/3$ cup
sheep's or goat's yogurt		2 tbsp	

Cook the onion in the oil, adding the green pepper halfway through until both are just softening. Add the chopped garlic, ginger and chilli and fry for 2 minutes. Add the turmeric, paprika and cinnamon and fry for a minute, then add the cooked chicken and stir well. (If fresh chicken chunks are used, add 150 ml/$1/4$ pt/$2/3$ cup water, cover and cook. Then reduce the liquid over a high heat, if necessary.) Stir in the coconut, cover and simmer over a medium heat until heated through. Add the yogurt and serve.

Serve with rice and salad or the vegetable curry on page 34.

SERVES 4

MARINATED ROAST CHICKEN BREASTS

This is good served with freshly picked sweetcorn and the Green Beans with Cherry Tomatoes on page 33. Chicken wings can also be used. After they have been marinated the chicken pieces can be barbecued instead of baked.

	METRIC	IMPERIAL	CUPS
6 chicken breasts/half breasts			
FOR THE MARINADE:			
French mustard		2 heaped tsp	
juice and grated rind of ½ lime			
juice and grated rind of ½ lemon			
chilli flakes		½ tsp	
balsamic vinegar		2 tbsp	
good tamari		5 tbsp	
maple syrup		1 tbsp	
2 large cloves garlic, very finely chopped/minced			
2.5 cm/1 in chopped fresh root ginger			
olive oil		2 tbsp	
black pepper			

Mix all the marinade ingredients together in a bowl. Cut 2 or 3 deep slashes across each chicken breast and submerge them in the mixture for at least an hour, or overnight.

Preheat the oven to 230°C/450°F/Gas 8.

Bake the chicken breasts in the marinade for 35 mintues. Finish under the grill/broiler for 3 minutes.

The marinade becomes a sauce, but you may need to pour off any excess oil and add a little water to moisten.

SERVES 6

LEMON TARRAGON CHICKEN WITH BUTTON MUSHROOMS

This is one of the most delicious ways to serve chicken. This dish should have a very fragrant smell from the tarragon and the sauce should be well flavoured with the lemon. Add more lemon or tarragon if necessary.

	METRIC	IMPERIAL	CUPS
1 chicken			
1 large sweet onion, finely chopped			
sunflower oil		3 tbsp	
button mushrooms	100 g	3 ½ oz	1 ½ cups
all-purpose wheat-free flour		4 tbsp	
chicken stock made during the poaching	1.2 litres	2 pints	5 cups
juice of at least 2 lemons			
black pepper			
1 large bunch fresh tarragon			

Preheat the oven to 180°C/350°F/Gas 4.

Place the chicken in a covered casserole with 1.2 litres/2 pints/5 cups water. Poach in the moderate oven for an hour or until the juices run clear when a skewer is jabbed into the thickest part of the thigh. Set aside to cool, reserving the stock for the sauce. This part can be prepared ahead of time and the sauce can be made at the last minute with the chicken chunks swiftly heated through.

Cook the onion in the oil in a heavy-bottomed casserole until it is clear and soft, but not coloured. Throw in the button mushrooms, sprinkle with the flour and mix. Remove from the heat and add the stock, lemon juice, plenty of freshly ground black pepper and the tarragon. Place back on a moderate heat and bring to the boil, stirring constantly until thickened. The sauce will take on a slightly greenish colour from the fresh tarragon.

Skin the chicken and remove the cooked meat from the bones. (The skin and bones can be made into stock, see page 155.) Cut the chicken into large chunks and put into the sauce. Heat through over a gentle heat, stirring.

Serve with rice or mashed potato with a green vegetable or a green salad.

SERVES 6

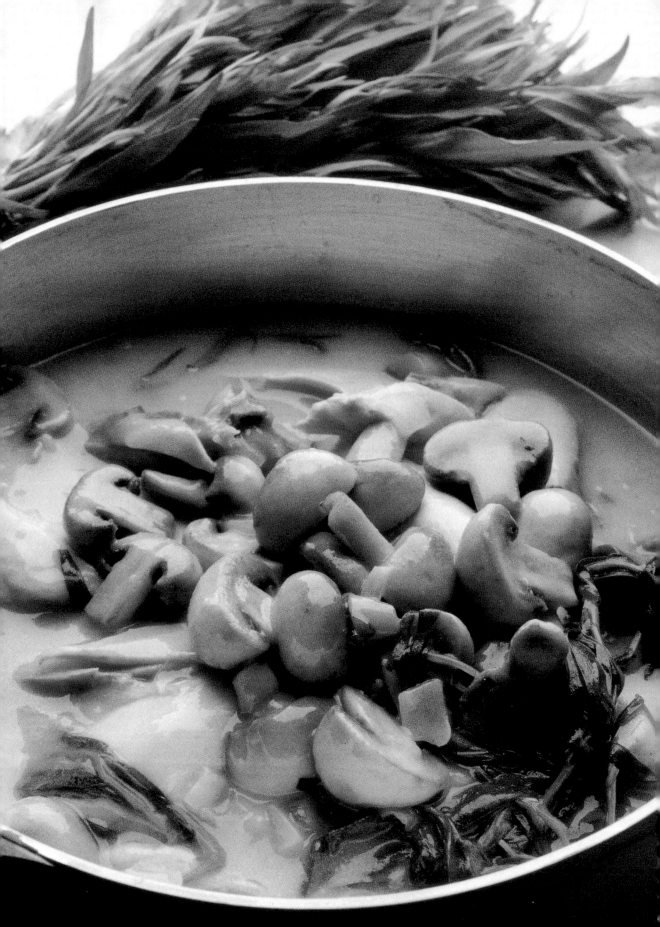

ROAST TURKEY THIGH WITH HONEY AND GINGER GLAZE

It is well worth marinating the turkey for 24 hours before cooking. Not only does the marinade permeate the meat, but it also tenderizes it. Leave the bone in the meat. This holds the thigh together during cooking and also adds flavour. The bone can be removed with a sharp knife before carving if you wish. The gravy made from the marinade and cooking juices is delicious. (Any leftovers can be made into Gougère or Shepherds' Pie, see pages 106 and 104.)

	METRIC	IMPERIAL	CUPS
turkey thigh, with the bone still in	900 g	2 lb	
arrowroot mixed with 1 tbsp water		2 tsp	
FOR THE MARINADE:			
Dijon mustard		½ tbsp	
good tamari		½ tbsp	
orange juice		1 tbsp	
ground ginger		1 tsp	
runny honey		1 tbsp	
olive oil		½ tbsp	
2 cloves garlic, crushed			

Mix all the marinade ingredients in a non-metallic bowl. Brush over both sides of the meat and leave for at least 2 hours, maximum 24 hours, before cooking. Cover and store in the refrigerator. Preheat the oven to 180°C/350°F/Gas 4. Put the meat in a roasting pan skin side down. Pour over any remaining marinade and put enough water in the roasting pan to cover the bottom by 6 mm/¼ in.

Allow 40 minutes' cooking time per 450 g/1 lb of turkey. Turn the turkey halfway through cooking and add a little more water to keep the bottom of the pan covered. When the cooking time has been completed, remove from the oven, place the meat on a serving dish and stand for 15 minutes before carving. Meanwhile, take the roasting pan and add enough liquid (stock or the water used for cooking the vegetables to accompany this meal) to make up to 300 ml/½ pt/1¼ cups of liquid. Scrape the residue and juices up from the pan and bring to the boil. Strain the gravy into a small saucepan, then return to the heat and adjust seasoning if necessary. Remove from the heat and stir in the arrowroot mixture to thicken the gravy.

Serve with two different vegetable purées such as carrot, squash or sweet potato with parsnip, celeriac/celery root or potato. These look pretty and are excellent for mopping up the delicious gravy.

SERVES 4–6

TURKEY BURGERS WITH SPICY TOMATO SAUCE

This is a quick and easy-to-make favourite. The sauce is good with a number of other dishes, including the potato fritters on page 62.

	METRIC	IMPERIAL	CUPS
raw turkey or chicken meat, minced/ground	675 g	1½ lb	
½ onion, grated			
1 egg, beaten			
seasoning to taste			
vegetable oil			
FOR THE SPICY TOMATO SAUCE:			
chilli flakes		½ tsp	
2 cloves garlic, crushed			
dried thyme		2 tsp	
olive oil		3 tbsp	
canned organic tomatoes	250 g	8½ oz	

Make the sauce first. Put the chilli flakes, garlic and thyme into the oil and gently fry for 1 minute. Add the tomatoes and simmer gently for 5 minutes. Keep warm.

For the burgers, mix the ingredients well and divide the mixture equally into 4. Form into patties with your hands. Fry the patties in vegetable oil, turning, until brown and cooked through, about 6–8 minutes each side depending on thickness. Test by piercing centre with a skewer. If juices run clear, then the burgers are cooked.

Serve with the spicy tomato sauce.

SERVES 4

'SHEPHERDS' PIE'

Traditionally, this is the way to use up cooked leftover lamb. Here cold turkey is substituted. The red vegetables – bell peppers, beans and tomatoes – give a lovely rich colour. The jalapeño chilli does not make the dish 'fiery' but just adds a depth of flavour.

	METRIC	IMPERIAL	CUPS
minced/ground cold cooked turkey	225 g	8 oz	2 cups
½ onion			
1 whole jalapeño chilli pepper, stalk removed			
olive oil		4 tbsp	
½ red bell pepper, cored, seeded and diced			
red kidney beans, cooked as per instructions on pack	175 g	6 oz	1 cup
canned tomatoes	400 g	14 oz	
tomato purée/paste		1 tbsp	
juice of ½ lemon			
black pepper			
3 potatoes, cooked and mashed			

Chop the onion and the jalapeño chilli together in an electric blender or chop finely with a sharp knife. Put the olive oil into a pan and start to cook the onion/chilli mixture over a medium heat. Add the diced red pepper to the onion mixture and cook until the onion is softened slightly but the red pepper is still crunchy. Add the minced turkey and stir. The meat will absorb the oil.

If using canned kidney beans, rinse thoroughly then drain. Drain the canned tomatoes, reserving the juice. Add the beans, tomatoes and tomato purée to the turkey mixture. Add enough of the tomato juice to moisten well. Add the lemon juice and pepper, cover and simmer until all the ingredients are cooked through, about 10–15 minutes. Preheat the oven to its hottest setting. Put the turkey mixture into a pie dish and cover with the mashed potato, smoothing the top. Make a wavy pattern on the potato using the rounded end of a spatula. To do this, firmly pat the end of the knife down the centre of the potatoes. Turn the dish round to face the other way. Now repeat the process making 2 lines of indentations either side of the centre line already made. Turn the dish again and repeat the process, making 2 lines of indentations on either side of the existing pattern. Repeat until all the potato is covered. Cook in the oven until the potato becomes crusty and golden, about 25–30 minutes.

SERVES 4

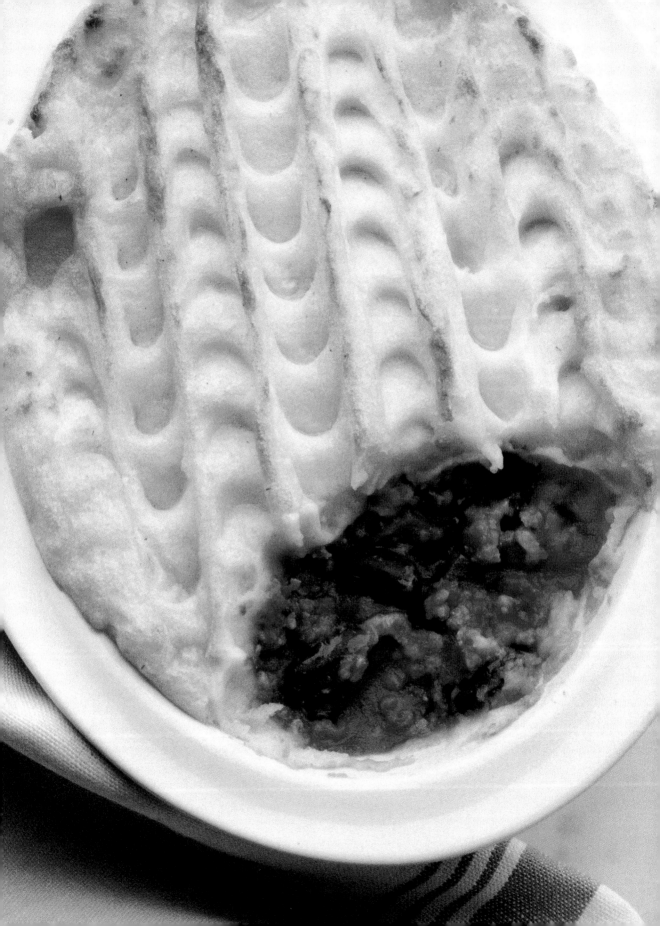

GOUGERE

This turns a very small amount of leftovers into a hearty supper. Use any leftover cooked meat that you may have: particularly delicious is the turkey with honey and ginger on page 102. Any vegetables can also be added. The thing to remember is that the mixture should be very highly flavoured and of a thick syrupy consistency. Omit the meat for a vegetarian option, which is equally delicious.

Do not be intimidated by the thought of making choux pastry. This recipe is foolproof provided a) the flour is sifted, b) the flour is added all at once off the heat and stirred only until the mixture leaves the sides of the pan and, c) enough egg mixture is added to make the mixture look smooth and glossy, but not too wet. Finally, make sure that the oven is well preheated.

	METRIC	IMPERIAL	CUPS
FOR THE FILLING:			
cooked turkey, chicken etc.	55–170 g	2–6 oz	⅓–1 cup
3 spring onions/scallions chopped into 1 cm/½ in slices			
olive oil		1 tbsp	
2 small flat mushrooms, sliced			
1 medium ripe tomato, roughly chopped, including skin if organic and seeds			
mixed dried herbs/Italian seasoning		1½ tsp	
2 cloves garlic, crushed			
tomato purée/paste, or sun-dried tomato purée/paste		1 tbsp	
plenty of black pepper			
FOR THE CHOUX PASTE:			
margarine	55 g	2 oz	¼ cup
water	150 ml	¼ pt	⅔ cup
all-purpose wheat-free flour, sifted	75 g	2½ oz	¾ cup
2 large eggs			
Dijon mustard		1 tsp	
black pepper			
goat's Cheddar cheese, diced into 6 mm/¼ in squares	115 g	4 oz	1 cup
goat's Cheddar cheese, coarsely grated	55 g	2 oz	½ cup

Preheat the oven to 220°C/425°F/Gas 7.

For the filling, put the onion, oil and mushrooms in a saucepan and cook over a medium heat for 2 minutes. Add the chopped tomato, herbs and crushed garlic and cook until the tomatoes have 'melted'. Add the tomato purée and pepper and stir. This mixture should be thick and shiny. If there is too much liquid, boil rapidly to reduce. Add the cooked meat, remove from the heat and leave to stand and absorb the flavours while you prepare the choux.

Bring the margarine and the water to the boil in a saucepan. As soon as the mixture reaches boiling point, remove from the heat and shoot in the sifted flour all at once. Stir thoroughly, but stop immediately the mixture comes away from the side of the pan. Set aside while you lightly oil a pie dish. In a bowl beat the eggs, to which you have added the mustard and pepper.

Vigorously stir the beaten eggs, a third at a time, into the flour mixture. It will look 'curdled' but will regain a smooth texture as you continue to beat. Do not overbeat. Stop as soon as the egg has been incorporated. Add more egg and continue the process until all the egg has been mixed in. The mixture should be smooth and shiny but not too wet. Add more or less of the egg mixture to achieve this consistency. Stir in the cheese cubes.

Put three-quarters of the mixture into the pie dish, bringing it up the sides with the back of a spoon. There should only be a very thin layer of paste in the centre of the pie dish. Spoon the filling into the centre of the dish. The choux paste around the sides should be higher than the filling mixture. Dollop the remaining choux paste over the top of the filling mixture. Spread this over the filling mixture, but do not cover it completely. The filling should appear in a gap between the choux on the edge of the pie dish and the choux topping.

Sprinkle with the grated cheese and bake in the hot oven for 45 minutes or until the choux is crisp, risen and golden.

SERVES 4

PHEASANT BRAISED WITH PLUMS

	METRIC	IMPERIAL	CUPS
1 pheasant			
plums	400 g	14 oz	
olive oil	60 ml	2 fl oz	¼ cup
sultanas	150 g	5 ½ oz	1 cup
2 dried bay leaves			
2 sprigs fresh thyme			
ground allspice		½ tsp	
lemon juice		1 tbsp	
balsamic vinegar		2 tbsp	
chopped celery	55 g	2 oz	½ cup
chopped leek	55 g	2 oz	½ cup
chicken stock (see page 155)	350 ml	12 fl oz	1 ½ cups

Preheat the oven to 180°C/350°F/Gas 4. Rinse the pheasant inside and out under cold running water. Pat dry with kitchen paper. In a flameproof casserole, heat the olive oil on the top of the stove. Brown the pheasant all over in the oil and set aside on a plate. Remove the casserole from the heat and add all the remaining ingredients. Stir well, scraping up any residue from the bottom. Return the bird to the casserole, breast down, cover and cook in the oven for 1 hour. Remove the casserole from the oven to turn the bird and stir the other ingredients. Cover, return to the oven and cook for another 30 minutes. By this time the bird should be cooked and the juices should run clean when a skewer is inserted into the thigh. If the bird is tough, cook for a further 30 minutes, covered.

Remove the bird from the casserole and place on a carving board. Remove the plum stones, bay leaves and thyme sprigs and put the contents of the casserole into a blender or food processor. Blend until smooth. Adjust seasoning to taste. Strain the sauce through a fine sieve back into the rinsed casserole, pressing the mixture through with a wooden spoon. If the mixture is too thick, add a little more stock. Carve off both of the legs and thighs from the bird and divide each into 2 pieces. Carve each side of the breast into 2 thick slices so you have 4 slices of breast and 4 pieces of leg. Return the pheasant to the casserole filled with the plum sauce. Reheat gently and serve. This is very good served with a purée made with celeriac/celery root and potatoes.

SERVES 4

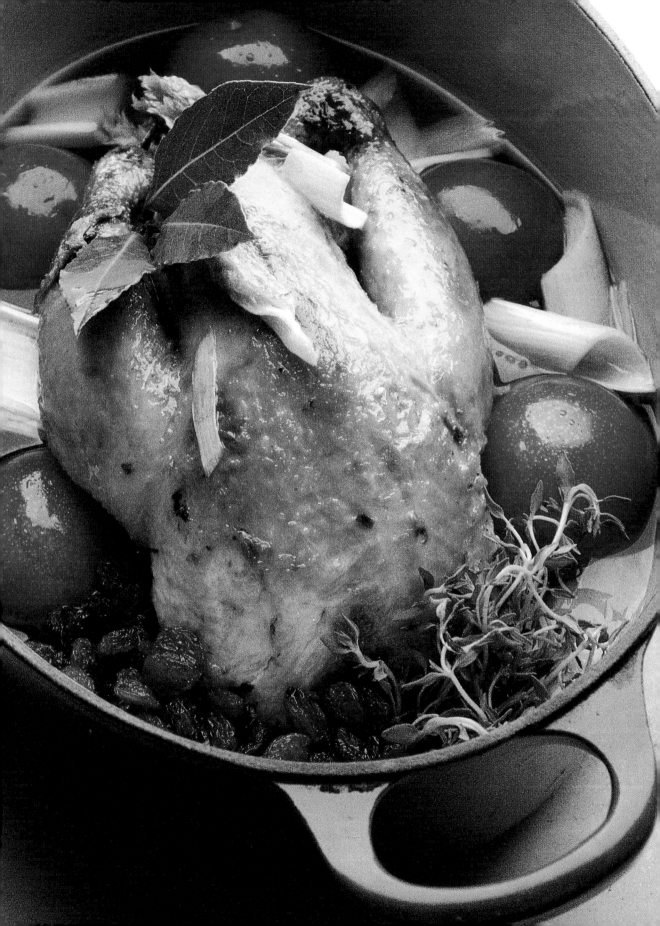

GREEN CHICKEN

This is a useful way to use leftover chicken and is delicious with rice, mashed potato or Parsnip and Garlic Mash (see page 42).

	METRIC	IMPERIAL	CUPS
olive oil		3 tbsp	
sunflower oil		1 tbsp	
1 large leek, including the green part, sliced			
mushrooms, sliced	200 g	7 oz	1 cup
chopped chives		5 tbsp	
juice of ½ lemon			
black pepper			
all-purpose wheat-free flour		4 tbsp	
soya milk	300 ml	½ pt	1¼ cups
chicken stock	300 ml	½ pt	1¼ cups
2 large cooked chicken breasts			

Heat the olive and sunflower oils in a casserole dish. Add the leek and cook until softened. Add mushrooms, chives, lemon juice and pepper and stir to combine. Stir in the flour to coat all ingredients, then add the soya milk and chicken stock, a little at a time, stirring. Bring to the boil and simmer gently for 5 minutes.

Add the chicken and heat through. The chicken breasts may be left whole or chopped into chunks – or you can use other leftover chicken pieces (but make sure that they are heated right through).

SERVES 2

GUINEA FOWL AND TURNIP

This dish may sound heavy but it is, in fact, very sweet and light. It is well worth using an organic turnip because the flavour is so much better.

	METRIC	IMPERIAL	CUPS
1 guinea fowl			
1 large turnip			
sunflower oil		3 tbsp	
olive oil		3 tbsp	
1 sprig fresh rosemary			
1 sprig fresh thyme			
3 whole cloves garlic			
white wine vinegar		½ tbsp	
black pepper			
lemon juice		½ tbsp	
water	300 ml	½ pt	1 ¼ cups
sheep's yogurt		4 tbsp	

Preheat the oven to 180°C/350°F/Gas 4.

Put the mixed oils into a flameproof casserole and heat on the top of the stove. Brown the bird on all sides and put aside on a plate. Peel and cut the turnip roughly into 5 cm/2 in cubes and toss in the oil. Put all the remaining ingredients apart from the yogurt – herbs, garlic, vinegar, black pepper, lemon juice and water – into the dish and place the guinea fowl on top. Cover and cook in the oven for 1 hour or until ready.

Place the turnips at one end of a serving dish and the carved and jointed bird at the other. Strain the juices into a saucepan, reducing if necessary, and stir in the yogurt. Pour the sauce over the guinea fowl and serve. (Use the carcass for stock, see page 155.)

SERVES 6–8

ROAST QUAILS WITH WILD RICE, PINE KERNELS AND APRICOT CAKES

American wild rice is a real treat. For years I followed the cooking instructions on the pack which call for long cooking times. Unfortunately this method causes the rice to split unevenly and lose its exquisite appearance. Follow these simple suggestions and your rice grains will retain their slender shape.

	METRIC	IMPERIAL	CUPS
4 quails			
a little sunflower oil			
FOR THE RICE CAKES:			
wild rice	110 g	3 ½ oz	⅔ cup
dried apricots	170 g	6 oz	
2 egg whites			
sweet onion, finely chopped	115 g	4 oz	scant 1 cup
zest of 1 lemon			
zest of 1 large orange			
pine kernels, toasted	55 g	2 oz	⅓ cup
black pepper			

Preheat the oven to 180°C/350°F/Gas 4. Put the wild rice and dried apricots into separate bowls, cover with boiling water and leave for 1 hour.

In a fine sieve, drain the rice and rinse under cold running water. Bring a pan of water to a vigorous boil, put in the rice and simmer for 10 minutes then drain. Drain the apricots and put 2 or 3 in the body cavity of each of the quails. Put the birds in a small roasting pan and brush the skin with a little oil.

In a mixing bowl, put the egg whites, broken with a fork but not whisked, the onion, the lemon and orange zests, the pine kernels, the cooked wild rice and the rest of the apricots roughly chopped. Mix the ingredients together well and add plenty of freshly milled black pepper. Roast the quails for 30–35 minutes. Meanwhile, lightly grease a baking sheet and the inside of 4 pancake rings. Divide the rice mixture evenly between the rings, smoothing and pressing down lightly with your knuckles. These will take 15 minutes to cook, so 15 minutes before the end of the roasting time, put the rice cakes into the oven. Place a rice cake on each plate with a quail on top. Serve with a salad of fresh watercress.

SERVES 4

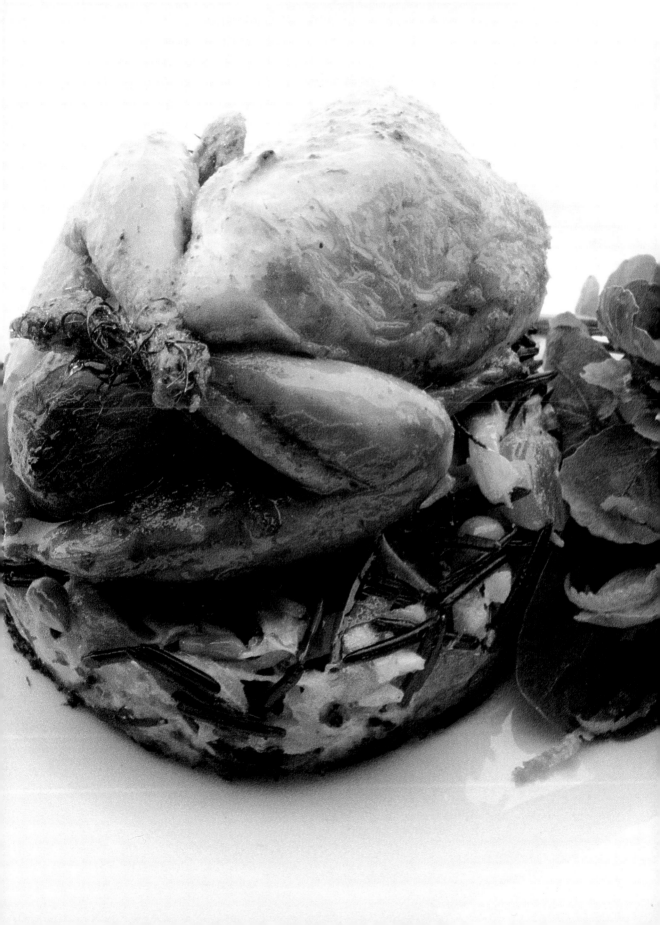

WILD DUCK BRAISED WITH FENNEL

Celery hearts can replace the fennel if preferred.

	METRIC	IMPERIAL	CUPS
1 wild duck			
sunflower oil		3 tbsp	
olive oil		2 tbsp	
2 fennel bulbs			
2 garlic cloves			
FOR THE MARINADE:			
Dijon mustard		1 tsp	
honey		2 tsp	
tamari		4 tbsp	
balsamic vinegar		2 tbsp	
blood orange juice	175 ml	6 fl oz	¾ cup
squeeze of lemon juice			
black pepper			

Preheat the oven to 190°C/375°F/Gas 5.

Heat the oils together in a flameproof casserole on the top of the stove and brown the duck on all sides. Remove and place on a plate. Trim the feathery leaves from the top of the fennel bulbs and keep to one side. Cut the fennel into quarters through the stem of the bulb which will hold the pieces together during cooking. Put in the casserole, add the garlic cloves and place the duck on top. Pour over the marinade, cover and cook in the oven for an hour or until the duck is cooked and the fennel is tender.

Cut the duck into quarters and place on a serving dish surrounded by the fennel. Pour over the juices, removing the garlic cloves, and adjust the seasoning to taste. Scissor over the feathery fennel leaves to garnish.

This is excellent served with a vegetable purée – potato, carrot, parsnip, acorn squash etc. – and a simple green salad.

SERVES 4

DUCK WITH SUN-DRIED TOMATOES AND CANNELLINI BEANS

This is a quick version of the French favourite, cassoulet. A hearty dish, ideal after a bracing winter walk.

	METRIC	IMPERIAL	CUPS
duck meat, cut into 2.5 cm/1 in cubes, skin removed	170–225 g	6–8 oz	1–1¼ cups
olive oil		2 tbsp	
caraway seeds		½ tsp	
2 cans cannellini beans, rinsed thoroughly and drained	2 x 425 g	2 x 14½ oz	
malt extract		½ tsp	
plenty of black pepper			
3 large cloves garlic, crushed			
1 big bunch fresh thyme			
chopped sun-dried tomatoes		4 tbsp	
oil from the sun-dried tomatoes		1 tbsp	
Dijon mustard		½ tsp	
water or stock (see page 155)	250 ml	8 fl oz	1 cup
1 x 7.5 cm/3 in piece unwaxed lemon peel			

Heat the olive oil in a flameproof casserole. When it is hot, put in the duck pieces and cook rapidly to seal. Stir in the caraway seeds and cook for 1 minute. Remove from the heat and stir in the rest of the ingredients – the beans, malt extract, pepper, garlic, thyme, tomatoes, their oil, mustard, stock and lemon peel. Return to the heat and bring slowly to the boil. Remove the lemon peel and save to use as a garnish. Turn down the heat and very gently simmer the stew, covered, for 30 minutes, stirring from time to time. Add more liquid if necessary. Remove stalks from the thyme, adjust seasoning to taste, and garnish with the lemon peel.

Serve with a green salad.

SERVES 3–4

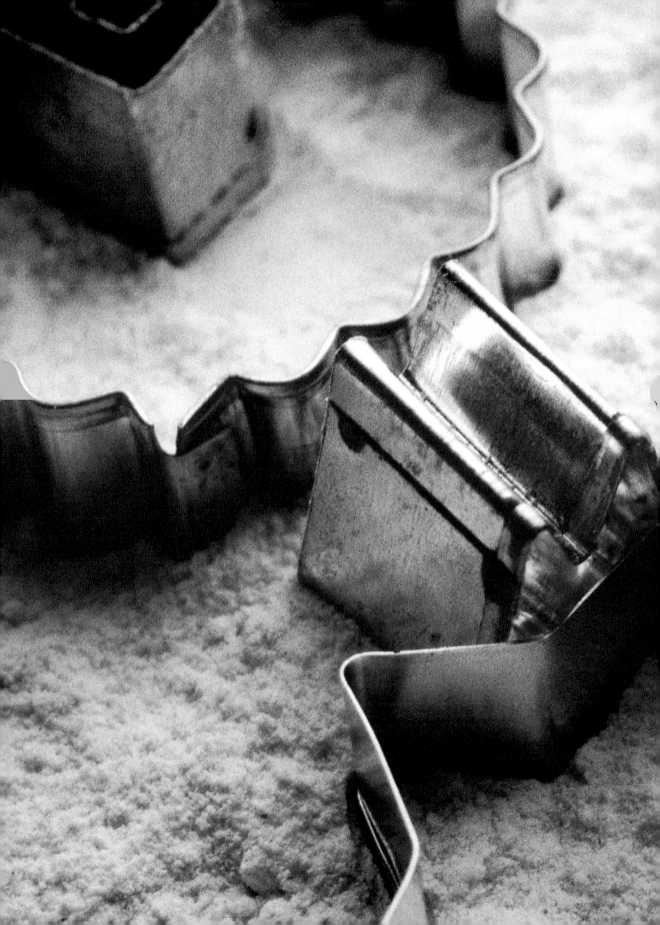

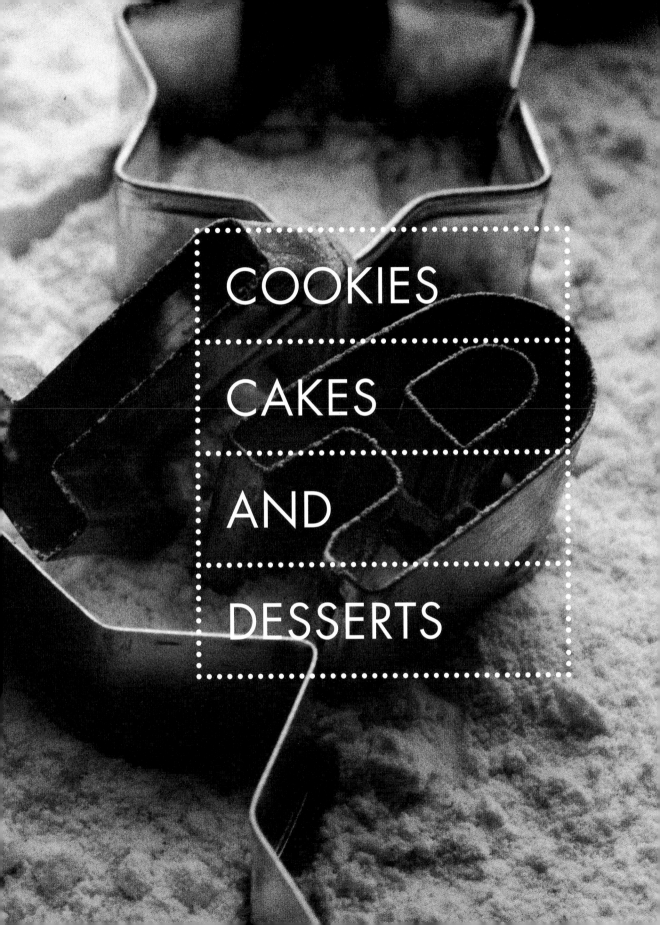

COOKIES

CAKES

AND

DESSERTS

ALMOND COOKIES

These crumbly little cookies melt in the mouth. They look very pretty and are ideal to serve with fresh fruit or with the Lemon Ice on page 143.

	METRIC	IMPERIAL	CUPS
all-purpose wheat-free flour	90 g	3 oz	scant 1 cup
ground almonds	30 g	1 oz	1/3 cup
margarine	75 g	2 1/2 oz	5 tbsp
fructose	30 g	1 oz	2 1/2 tbsp
almond extract		1 tsp	
1 egg, beaten			
flaked almonds	55 g	2 oz	1/2 cup

Put the flour, ground almonds, margarine and fructose into a food processor with the blade attachment and pulse until the mixture resembles crumbs. Add the almond extract and 2 tbsp of the beaten egg. As soon as the dough forms a ball, take it out. Knead slightly. The dough will be soft and slightly sticky. Roll into a ball, wrap and refrigerate for at least 1 hour.

Preheat the oven to 160°C/325°F/Gas 3.

Flour a surface and a rolling pin and roll the dough out as thinly as possible. Using a pastry brush lightly coat the surface of the dough with the remaining egg. Sprinkle over the flaked almonds and roll in lightly with the rolling pin. Cut with a cookie cutter and carefully arrange on a baking sheet.

Bake for 15 minutes until a light golden brown. Do not allow to darken.

Cool on a wire rack.

MAKES 12–15 SMALL COOKIES

SESAME SEED AND CHERRY HONEY SQUARES

Any dried fruits can be substituted for the cherries, and any choice of seeds or nuts can replace the sesame seeds. The tartness of the cherries combined with the toasted sesame seeds makes this recipe a favourite with family and friends – and it could not be simpler to make. These squares are special enough to serve as dessert with fresh fruit salad or a bowl of fresh fruits.

	METRIC	IMPERIAL	CUPS
margarine	115 g	4 oz	½ cup
runny honey		3 tbsp	
porridge oats	115 g	4 oz	scant 1 cup
jumbo rolled oats	30 g	1 oz	scant ¼ cup
dried cherries	90 g	3 oz	
sesame seeds	90 g	3 oz	⅔ cup

Preheat the oven to 180°C/350°F/Gas 4.

In a saucepan, melt the margarine and the honey until bubbling. Boil for about 1 minute but be careful that the mixture does not darken. Off the heat, shoot all the oats in at once and stir. Then add the rest of the ingredients and mix well. Return the mixture to the heat and cook, stirring, for a minute or two.

Lightly oil a shallow tin approximately 15 cm/6 in square. Fill with the mixture, pressing it firmly down with the back of a spoon. Place in the middle of the preheated oven and cook for about 30 minutes or until golden brown all over.

Remove from the oven and pack the mixture down firmly once again and mark out into 9 squares. Cool on a wire rack and then refrigerate until completely cold. Take care when removing the first square and then the rest can be easily removed from the tin with a spatula. Store in an airtight container.

MAKES 9 SQUARES

FRESH GINGER AND HONEY COOKIES WITH PINE KERNELS

These ginger cookies are very crisp.

	METRIC	IMPERIAL	CUPS
fine oatmeal flour	55 g	2 oz	scant ¹/₂ cup
all-purpose wheat-free flour	55 g	2 oz	¹/₂ cup
pine kernels		2¹/₂ tbsp	
grated fresh root ginger		3 tbsp	
runny honey		2 tbsp	
baking powder		¹/₈ tsp	
sunflower oil		1¹/₂ tbsp	

Preheat the oven to 150°C/300°F/Gas 2.

Put all the ingredients into a mixing bowl and gather together with your hands to form a ball. Kneed the mixture in the bowl until it is smooth. The mixture will start out feeling rather wet, but as the flour absorbs the honey and oil, the dough with become firmer. It should look very glossy and have no cracks at all. If necessary, add some more oil to moisten.

Pinch out enough dough to form balls of about the size of a walnut and place these balls on an ungreased baking sheet, 7.5 cm/3 in apart. Using the heel of your thumb and palm, flatten the balls of dough as thinly as possible. This can also be done using a metal spatula. Tuck any loose edges of the mixture back into the dough to form a circular cookie.

Bake for 20 minutes or until evenly golden and cooked thoroughly. Cool on a wire rack.

MAKES ABOUT 8 COOKIES

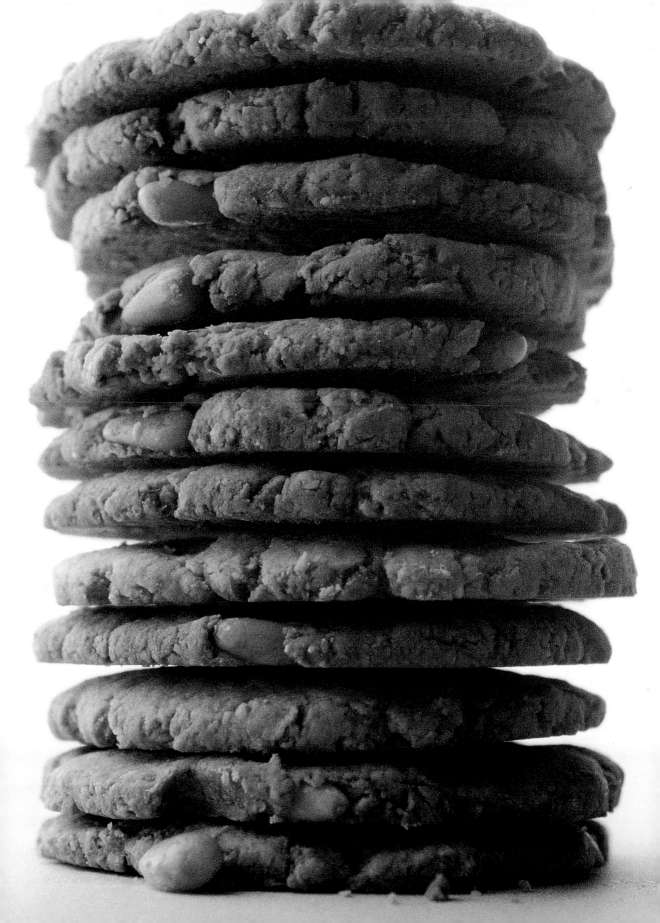

CHEESE TRIANGLES

These crumbly little biscuits are ideal to serve with drinks, soups or salads. They are very easy to make and the dough can be frozen.

	METRIC	IMPERIAL	CUPS
all-purpose wheat-free flour	115 g	4 oz	1 1/4 cups
grainy mustard		1/2 tsp	
cayenne pepper		1/4 tsp	
turmeric		1/4 tsp	
margarine, diced	75 g	2 1/2 oz	5 tbsp
hard cheese (e.g. goat's Cheddar), grated	55 g	2 oz	1/2 cup
pecorino cheese, grated	15 g	1/2 oz	1 tbsp
1 egg yolk			
cold water		2–3 tsp	

Preheat the oven to 180°C/350°F/Gas 4.

Put the flour, mustard and spices into a bowl, and cut in the margarine, blending with the tips of your fingers until the mixture resembles crumbs. Add the cheeses, and toss lightly to mix. Add the egg yolk and enough water to make a stiff paste. The amount of water needed will vary according to the moisture of the cheese and the size of the yolk. Knead until smooth and crack free. The mixture will look and feel rather like marzipan/almond paste. Form into a ball.

The dough can also be made in a food processor using the blade. Put the flour, spices, margarine and cheeses into the processor and pulse to coarse crumbs. Add the yolk and enough water by degrees until the dough forms a smooth ball.

Wrap and refrigerate for 20 minutes. Roll out on a floured surface to a thickness of about 6mm/1/4 in. Cut the dough in horizontal slices 3.5 cm/1 1/2 in wide and cut these slices into triangles. Place on a lightly floured baking tray and bake for 15–20 minutes. Cool on a wire rack.

MAKES ABOUT 4 DOZEN TRIANGLES

SCOTTISH OATCAKES WITH SESAME SEEDS

This recipe uses neither salt nor sweetener so the oatcakes taste equally good with cheeses, honey and jams. They keep very well in an airtight container.

	METRIC	IMPERIAL	CUPS
sesame seeds	15 g	1/2 oz	
fine oatmeal	115 g	4 oz	
jumbo oats	15 g	1/2 oz	
bicarbonate of soda/baking soda		1/8 tsp	
warm water		6 tbsp	
sunflower oil		1 tbsp	

Preheat the oven to 180°C/350°F/Gas 4. Place the sesame seeds on a baking tray and bake until just turning a golden brown. Cool.

Mix with all the remaining ingredients in a bowl and stir with your hands to form a ball. The mixture will feel wet and sticky to begin with but as the oats absorb the water and oil the mixture will stiffen. Knead for a few minutes to form a smooth dough. The dough must be crack free. If cracks appear now or when you are rolling out the mixture, break the dough up into pieces, put it back into the bowl and add more water to moisten and reform into a ball.

Using more of the fine oatmeal, dust a surface and a rolling pin, and roll out the mixture as thin as possible. Using a 5 cm/2 in cookie cutter, cut into circles and place the oatcakes on a baking sheet without oiling it.

Bake at the above temperature for 15 minutes, then turn and bake for a further 5 minutes or until the edges start to colour and the oatcakes are crisp and dry through.

These oatcakes can be eaten hot straight from the oven.

MAKES ABOUT 15 OATCAKES

DATE AND WALNUT MUFFINS WITH ORANGE ZEST AND NUTMEG

These muffins are light and crumbly and easy to make.

The margarine used in this recipe is a kosher variety which sets firm in the refrigerator, is made from vegetable oils and contains no whey. I would suggest that you buy whole dates, then chop them at home. This is because the ready chopped variety are often rolled in sugar, whereas whole dates usually only have a light coating of vegetable oil. Fresh dates can also be used.

	METRIC	IMPERIAL	CUPS
all-purpose wheat-free flour	250g	8oz	2½ cups
baking powder		2½ tsp	
½ fresh nutmeg, finely grated			
hard margarine	100 g	3½ oz	7 tbsp
fructose	75g	2½ oz	⅓ cup
1 medium egg			
sheep's or goat's yogurt	300 ml	½ pt	1¼ cups
water	60 ml	2 fl oz	¼ cup
dates, chopped	175 g	6 oz	1 cup
shelled walnuts, chopped	55 g	2 oz	½ cup
zest of 1 orange			

Preheat the oven to 190°C/375°F/Gas 5.

Sift the flour and baking powder into a mixing bowl. Add the nutmeg. Using 2 knives, cut the margarine (which has come straight from the refrigerator) into the flour as if you were making pastry. When the margarine is in small pieces, rub in lightly using your fingertips until the mixture resembles crumbs. Stir in the fructose.

In a small mixing bowl, beat the egg, yogurt and water together lightly. Add the egg mixture to the flour mixture and fold in with a metal spoon. Add the chopped dates, walnuts and orange zest and mix well. The mixture will be stiff. Spoon into paper muffin cases and place in a muffin pan. Smooth the tops slightly, then bake for 20 minutes.

MAKES 10 MUFFINS

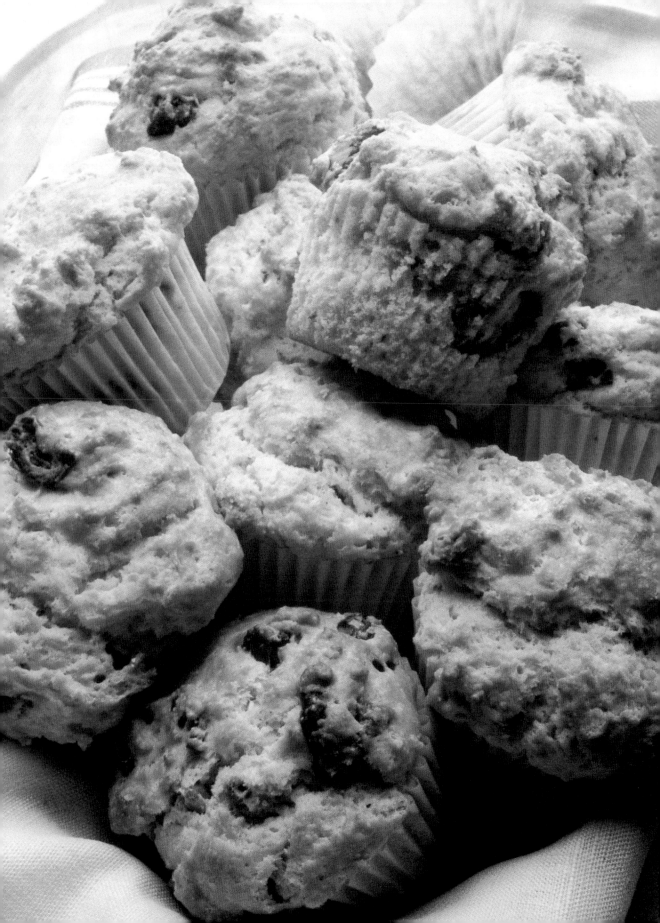

SCOTCH PANCAKES

One afternoon when having tea with Terence Stamp, he started to reminisce about the wonderful scotch pancakes that his mother used to make. We donned aprons and in a jiffy made up a batch of these pancakes. They could not be simpler and are great fun to make!

For American-style breakfast pancakes, simply drop larger spoonfuls of batter into the pan. You may also like to add blueberries, or raisins that have been soaked for a few minutes in boiling water.

	METRIC	IMPERIAL	CUPS
all-purpose wheat-free flour	225 g	8 oz	2¼ cups
bicarbonate of soda/baking soda		½ tsp	
cream of tartar		½ tsp	
baking powder		½ tsp	
soya milk	300 ml	½ pt	1¼ cups
1 egg			
sunflower oil		2 tbsp	
a pinch of salt			
runny honey or agave syrup		4 tbsp	¼ cup
vanilla extract		2 tsp	

Sieve the flour, bicarbonate of soda, cream of tartar and baking powder into a large mixing bowl. Make a well in the centre and whisk in most of the soya milk. Break the egg into the batter and add the oil, salt, honey or syrup and vanilla extract. Whisk in well to mix thoroughly.

Let the batter stand for 5 minutes, then gently stir in remaining soya milk if the mixture is too thick. (It should have the consistency of very thick cream, but be runny enough to pour off the back of a spoon.)

Heat a lightly greased frying pan/skillet, removing any excess oil with a piece of kitchen towel. Drop large spoonfuls of the batter, a few at a time, into the hot pan. When bubbles appear and burst, turn the pancakes and cook them on the other side for a minute or two until firm and cooked through. Repeat until all the mixture is used up.

MAKES 12–16 PANCAKES

HIGH TEA FRUIT CAKE

Terence Stamp's mother always cooked a rich fruit cake for Christmas. Family tradition had it that everyone was involved in choosing the ingredients, and the rich taste is one of Terence's most vivid childhood memories. Terence loves allspice, which his friend, Alice, grows in her garden in Hawaii. Even the leaves smell wondrous!

	METRIC	IMPERIAL	CUPS
orange juice	150 ml	1/4 pt	2/3 cup
dried yeast	7 g	1/4 oz	
all-purpose wheat-free flour	160 g	5 3/4 oz	1 2/3 cups
ground allspice		1 tsp	
ground ginger		1/2 tsp	
ground cinnamon		1/2 tsp	
grated nutmeg		1/2 tsp	
ground almonds	75 g	2 1/2 oz	1/2 cup
sunflower oil		3 tbsp	
dessert apple, cored but not peeled if organic	90 g	3 oz	
carrot, scrubbed and chopped	55 g	2 oz	1/2 cup
dried mixed fruit	225 g	8 oz	1 1/4 cups
zest of 1 unwaxed lemon			
zest of 1 unwaxed orange			
whole almonds to decorate (optional)	55 g	2 oz	1/2 cup

Preheat the oven to 180°C/350°F/Gas 4. Warm the orange juice in a saucepan. When lukewarm pour into a food processor and sprinkle over the yeast. Leave to soften for a few minutes.

Sift the flour and all the spices into a bowl, then stir in the ground almonds. Add the oil and stir.

Add the apple and carrot to the yeast and juice in the food processor and blend, leaving the apple and carrot in small pieces. Stir into the flour and oil mixture. Stir in the dried fruit and lemon and orange zests.

Lightly oil a 18 cm/7 in round cake tin. Line the base with a circle of greaseproof paper/baking parchment. Pour the cake mixture into the tin. Decorate with the almonds and bake for 1 hour or until a skewer inserted in the centre comes out cleanly. Cool in the pan. Remove the cake and wrap in foil to store or place in an airtight tin.

SERVES 8

CHOCOLATE CAKE WITH ROASTED HAZELNUTS

Anyone who doubts that a featherlight cake can be made without wheat flour should try this!

	METRIC	IMPERIAL	CUPS
hazelnuts, skinned, roasted and lightly crushed	100 g	4 oz	³/₄ cup
margarine	225 g	8 oz	1 cup
vanilla extract		2 tsp	
almond extract		2 tsp	
unsweetened cocoa powder		4 tbsp	
fructose	200 g	7 oz	1 cup
4 medium eggs			
all-purpose wheat-free flour	100 g	3¹/₂ oz	1 cup
baking powder		1 tsp	
FOR THE FROSTING:			
margarine	225 g	8 oz	1 cup
vanilla extract		³/₄ tsp	
unsweetened cocoa powder, sifted		12 tbsp	
maple syrup		1¹/₂ tbsp	

Preheat the oven to 180°C/350°F/Gas 4. In a saucepan, melt the margarine with the vanilla and almond extracts and sifted cocoa powder until just melted. Do not boil. Stir and remove from the heat. In a mixing bowl, beat the fructose into the eggs until they become light and thick, using a balloon whisk or electric mixer. Do this thoroughly to achieve lightness in the finished sponge. Stir in the margarine mixture. Sift the flour and baking powder into the mixture and stir. Add the nuts and mix well.

Cut two circles of greaseproof paper/baking parchment and place in the bottom of two 25 cm/10 in round cake tins. Divide the mixture evenly between the two tins and bake for 20 minutes. The sponges will seem soft when removed from the oven and will come away from the sides of the tins if pulled gently with your fingers. Allow to cool for 5 minutes and then turn out on two wire racks to cool.

Put all the frosting ingredients into a mixing bowl and using a balloon whisk or electric mixer, beat until thoroughly blended. Refrigerate until the cakes have completely cooled. To assemble the cake, put one of the cakes bottom side up on an upturned plate. Cover with a layer of frosting. Then place the other cake on top, bottom side down and frost the top and sides. Refrigerate until time to serve.

SERVES 8

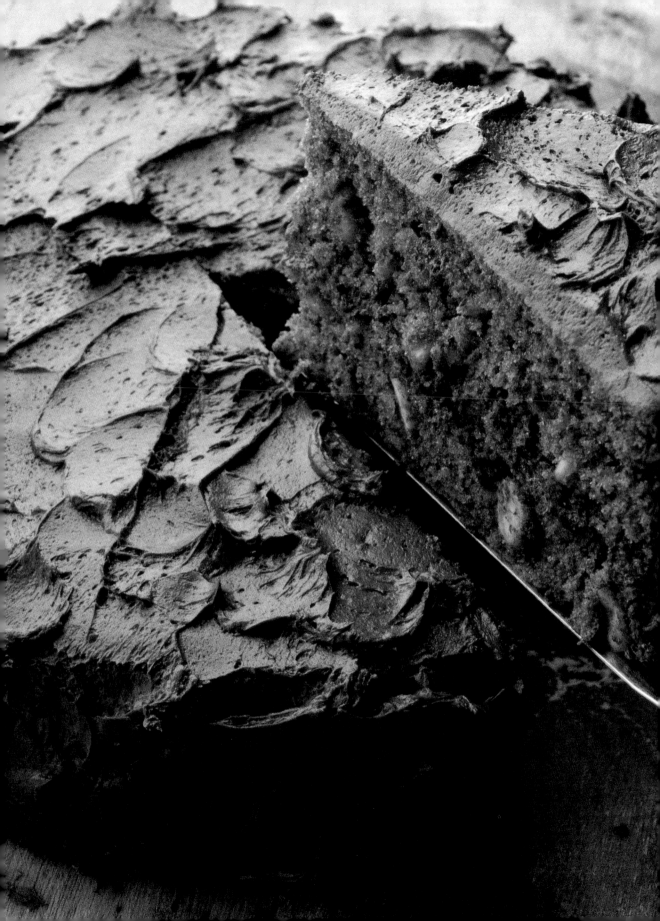

DOUBLE-CRUSTED NECTARINE PIE

	METRIC	IMPERIAL	CUPS
FOR THE PASTRY:			
all-purpose wheat-free flour	225 g	8 oz	2¼ cups
hard vegetable margarine	115 g	4 oz	1 cup
2 eggs			
FOR THE NECTARINE FILLING:			
6 large nectarines			
cornflour/cornstarch		1 tbsp	
fructose	200 g	7 oz	1 cup
ground cinnamon		1 tsp	
FOR THE GLAZE:			
1 egg, lightly beaten with 1 tbsp water			

Preheat the oven to 200°C/400°F/Gas 6.

Sift the flour into a bowl and cut in the margarine. Using your fingertips, rub in lightly until the mixture resembles fine breadcrumbs. Beat the egg with 1 tbsp cold water. Sprinkle this over the crumb mixture and mix lightly. This should form a pliable but not sticky dough. Wrap and refrigerate while preparing the nectarine filling.

Slice the nectarines into fairly large segments, removing the stones/pits. Place segments into a large mixing bowl and add the flour, fructose and cinnamon. Mix thoroughly.

Roll out half the pastry to line a 18 cm/7 in pie plate. Prick well with a fork. Fill with the nectarine mixture, piling it high in the middle. Roll out the remaining pastry and place on top of the fruit. Dampen between the two pieces of pastry with the egg glaze mixture to seal. Press the edges together firmly, trim and decorate with a fork. Make a steam hole in the centre of the pastry and decorate with leaves made from the pastry trimmings. Brush with egg glaze and bake for 30 minutes or until the pastry is golden brown.

SERVES 4

MAPLE SYRUP AND SULTANA SCONES

We have received dozens of requests for a simple scone recipe, so here it is!

	METRIC	IMPERIAL	CUPS
all-purpose wheat-free flour	170 g	6 oz	1 ¾ cups
baking powder		1 tbsp	
bicarbonate of soda/baking soda		½ tsp	
hard margarine	55 g	2 oz	¼ cup
goat's or sheep's milk		1 tbsp	
maple syrup		4 tbsp	¼ cup
sultanas/golden raisins	55 g	2 oz	⅓ cup
1 egg, beaten			

Sift the flour, baking powder and bicarbonate of soda together into a mixing bowl. Rub in the margarine until the mixture resembles crumbs. Add the milk, maple syrup and sultanas and stir to make a sticky paste. Let stand for 15 minutes to absorb liquids. Meanwhile, preheat the oven to 230°C/450°F/Gas 8.

Knead mixture into a soft dough. Roll out on a floured surface and cut into rounds using a 5cm/2in cookie cutter. Brush with beaten egg and bake for 10 minutes, until lightly golden.

MAKES 8 SCONES

CARROT, PINEAPPLE AND WALNUT CAKE

This is one of my daughter Poppy's recipes. Poppy has a very sweet tooth and learnt at a young age to bake cookies and cakes. I much prefer fresh fruit to finish off a meal, but Poppy pleaded for cakes. So we donned our aprons, got out the mixing bowls and the wooden spoons and have baked together since she was three years old. By the time Poppy was eight, she was baking goods for a friend's sandwich shop. The words 'Poppy Buxton's Chocolate Cake', written boldly in chalk on the menu board, justifiably made her pleased and proud. It was about this time that Terence Stamp heard about Poppy's baking skills and asked her to bake him a cake. When it was ready, Terence came to collect the cake and thus entered our lives to become a friend of all the family.

	METRIC	IMPERIAL	CUPS
FOR THE CAKE:			
4 large eggs			
fructose	150 g	5½ oz	¾ cup
vegetable oil	125 ml	4 fl oz	½ cup
all-purpose wheat-free flour	200 g	7 oz	2 cups
baking powder		2 tsp	
bicarbonate of soda/baking soda		½ tsp	
ground cinnamon		2 tbsp	
ground ginger		¼ tsp	
carrot, grated	180 g	6½ oz	2 heaped cups
pineapple canned in juice (retain the juice), chopped	225 g	8 oz	2¼ cups
walnut pieces	115 g	4 oz	1 cup
vanilla extract		2 tsp	
FOR THE FROSTING (optional):			
fructose	225 g	8 oz	1⅛ cups
a little pineapple juice (see above)			
lemon juice and vanilla extract		1 tsp each	
margarine	170 g	6 oz	¾ cup
goat's cream cheese	170 g	6 oz	¾ cup

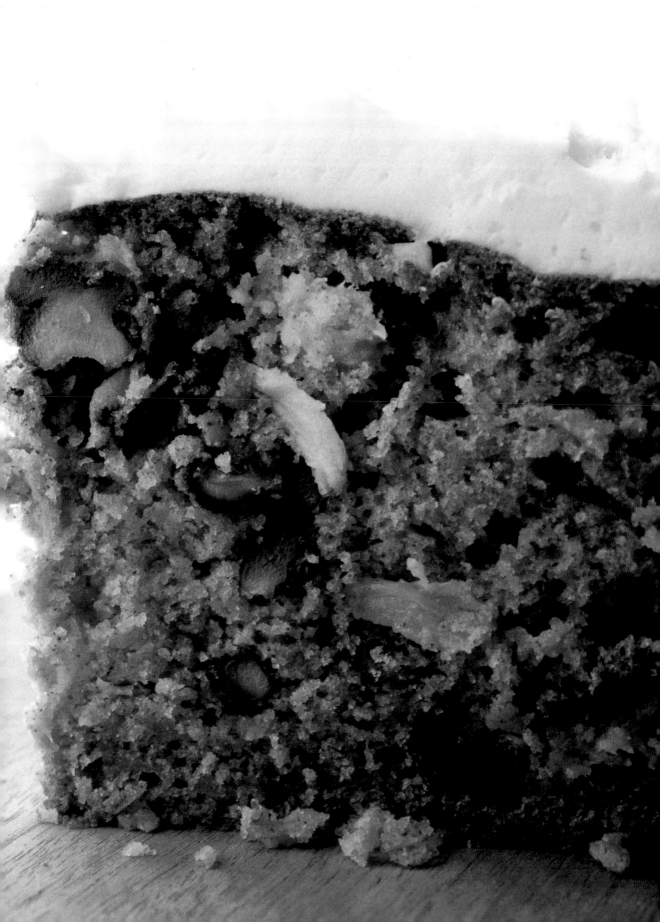

CARROT, PINEAPPLE AND WALNUT CAKE continued

Preheat the oven to 180°C/350°F/Gas 4.

Beat the eggs well, add the fructose and oil and continue to beat. Sift in the flour, baking powder, bicarbonate of soda, cinnamon and ginger. Continue to beat until thoroughly mixed. Stir in the carrot, pineapple, walnuts and vanilla extract. Pour into a lightly oiled 20 cm/8 in round non-stick cake tin and bake for 40–45 minutes. The cake should be just firm and have come away from the side of the tin slightly. Do not overbake.

Remove from the oven and allow to cool for 10 minutes, then turn out and cool completely on a wire rack before frosting.

Put the fructose, pineapple juice, lemon juice and vanilla extract into a small saucepan and dissolve, shaking it in a circular motion. When the mixture starts to bubble, lift the pan and hold it above the heat. Allow to bubble further for a few seconds to form a thick syrup. Remove from the heat before the syrup colours, and set aside to cool completely.

In a bowl or food processor, mix the margarine and cream cheese. Add 2 tbsp of the syrup and mix well. Chill until needed, then spread on the top of the cake with a spatula.

SERVES 8

FRUIT CLAFOUTIS

Any ripe, soft seasonal fruit can be used for the base: pears, peaches, nectarines, plums or a mixture of your choice. Here we have used Terence Stamp's favourite mixed berries.

	METRIC	IMPERIAL	CUPS
2 punnets blackberries			
1 punnet redcurrants, stalks removed			
1 punnet blueberries			
1 punnet raspberries			
2 punnets strawberries, hulled and cut in half lengthways			
fructose		2 tbsp	
a little vegetable oil			
toasted almond flakes			
FOR THE TOPPING:			
all-purpose wheat-free flour	50 g	2 oz	1/2 cup
ground almonds	100 g	3 1/2 oz	1 1/2 cups
fructose	200 g	7 oz	1 cup
bicarbonate of soda/baking soda		1 tsp	
4 eggs			
sunflower oil	250 g	8 fl oz	1 cup
almond extract		2–3 tsp	
vanilla extract		1 tsp	
zest of 1/2 lemon			

Preheat the oven to 190°C/375°F/Gas 5.

Lightly oil a large shallow ovenproof dish. Place the fruit in it, finishing with a layer of strawberries, cut side down. Sprinkle with the fructose.

For the topping sift all the dry ingredients into a bowl. Roughly beat the eggs into the oil and stir into the dry ingredients. Add the extracts and lemon zest, then pour evenly over the fruit.

Bake for 45 minutes or until set. (If the top is browning too much, cover loosely with foil for the remaining cooking time.) Sprinkle with toasted almonds. Serve warm or chilled with sheep's yogurt and fructose on the side.

SERVES 8

FRENCH PLUM TART WITH ALMOND PASTRY

	METRIC	IMPERIAL	CUPS
Crème Pâtissière (see page 152)			
almond extract		1 tsp	
12 ripe plums			
fructose		1 1/2 tbsp	
ground cinnamon		1/2 tsp	
bramble jelly (see page 147)		2 tbsp	
water		1 tbsp	
FOR THE PASTRY:			
all-purpose wheat-free flour	170 g	6 oz	1 3/4 cups
finely ground blanched almonds	55 g	2 oz	3/4 cup
hard margarine, cut into pieces	115 g	4 oz	1/2 cup
almond extract		1 tsp	
fructose	15 g	1/2 oz	
cold water		4 tbsp	

To make the pastry/dough, put the flour, ground almonds, margarine and fructose into a food processor with the blade. Pulse a couple of times until the mixture resembles crumbs. Add the almond extract and water and run the motor until a ball has formed. The pastry should be soft and smooth, with no cracks. Wrap and refrigerate for 1 hour. Make the crème pâtissière following the quantities and method on page 152, but replacing the vanilla extract with 1 tsp almond extract. Refrigerate. Preheat the oven to 180°C/350°F/Gas 4. Cut the plums in half and remove the stones/pits. Place skin side down on a lightly oiled baking sheet and sprinkle with the fructose and cinnamon. Place the plums in the preheated oven for 15 minutes or until just softening but not losing their shape. Set aside to cool. Turn the oven up to 190°C/375°F/Gas 5.

Roll out the pastry and line a rectangular tart tin. Press the pastry up the sides of the tin and into the corners. Prick the base with a fork. Place in the preheated oven for 10–15 minutes until the pastry is a light golden colour then set aside. Put the bramble jelly and water into a small saucepan and melt. While the tart case is still warm, carefully brush the inside of the pastry with the liquid jelly, using a pastry brush. Carefully spoon the cold crème pâtissière into the tart case, then arrange the plums on top, skin side up. Brush all over with the rest of the bramble jelly. Refrigerate until time to serve.

SERVES 6

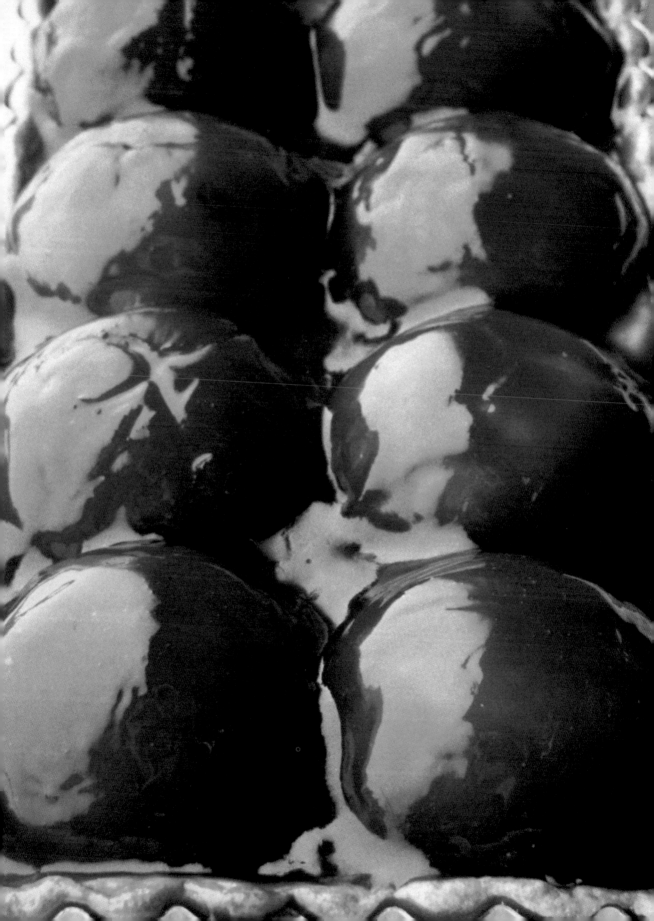

BANANA AND RHUBARB CRUMBLE

The flavour of bananas is accentuated when they are cooked. They add a depth and sweetness to another favourite – rhubarb crumble. If you prefer to use only rhubarb, then double its quantities. We have used jumbo rolled oats and ground almonds in the crumble which also add flavour and texture.

	METRIC	IMPERIAL	CUPS
rhubarb	325 g	11 oz	
fructose	55 g	2 oz	1/4 cup
4 small bananas, peeled			
FOR THE CRUMBLE:			
jumbo rolled oats	45 g	1 1/2 oz	1/2 cup
ground almonds	45 g	1 1/2 oz	1/3 cup
fructose	30 g	1 oz	1/8 cup
margarine	30 g	1 oz	2 tbsp

Preheat the oven to 190°C/375°F/Gas 5.

Put the oats, ground almonds and fructose into a bowl. Cut the margarine into the mixture in small pieces. Using your fingertips, lightly break the margarine into the other ingredients as if you were making pastry. Set aside.

Rinse the rhubarb and dry. Cut into 2.5 cm/1 in slices and put into a mixing bowl with the fructose. Stir. Cut the bananas into 1 cm/1/2 in chunks and mix into the rhubarb and fructose mixture.

Place the fruit in an ovenproof dish. Sprinkle over the crumble topping and bake for 30 minutes.

Serve with custard or yogurt.

SERVES 4

BANANA AND CINNAMON LOAF

One of the lovely things about working with the Stamp Collection is all the feedback that we get from customers. We receive dozens of telephone calls, emails, faxes and letters a day, and from these I have learnt a lot about the difficulties that people have overcoming their food intolerances and adjusting to wheat- and dairy-free diets. People also share their favourite recipes with us; here is one adapted from a recipe that was kindly sent to us by Sally Shepherd.

	METRIC	IMPERIAL	CUPS
all-purpose wheat-free flour	200 g	7 oz	2 cups
wheat-free baking powder		2 tsp	
bicarbonate of soda/baking soda		½ tsp	
ground cinnamon		1 tsp	
margarine	75 g	2½ oz	⅓ cup
4 large ripe bananas (the browner the better – the taste is stronger)			
agave syrup	75 ml	2½ fl oz	⅓ cup
2 eggs			

Preheat the oven to 180°C/350°F/Gas 4.

In a bowl, sift together flour, baking powder, bicarbonate of soda and cinnamon. Rub in the margarine to resemble crumbs. Mash 2 of the bananas with the agave syrup to form a runny purée and add to the bowl. Mash the other 2 bananas lightly (so that they are in small pieces) and add to the other ingredients. Beat the eggs, add them to the bowl and mix all ingredients together. Alternatively, put all ingredients in a food processor and process.

Grease a 900 g/2 lb loaf tin with margarine. Turn the mixture into it and bake in the preheated oven for 1 hour.

Turn the loaf out on to a wire rack to cool, then store in an airtight container.

This loaf can be eaten on its own or with margarine or cream cheese.

SERVES 8

STEAMED BLACKBERRY PUDDING

This is the ultimate comfort food. This recipe has several advantages: the sponge is light without losing that special 'steamed pudding' texture, and only egg whites are used in the sponge batter leaving 3 yolks to make custard to serve with the pudding.

	METRIC	IMPERIAL	CUPS
blackberries	170 g	6 oz	
fructose	115 g	4 oz	½ cup
margarine (use the soft variety)	90 g	3 oz	6 tbsp
mixture of half goat's milk and half sheep's yogurt	150 ml	¼ pt	⅔ cup
all-purpose wheat-free flour	170 g	6 oz	1¾ cups
baking powder		1 tbsp	
vanilla extract		1 tsp	
zest of 1 lemon			
3 egg whites			
Custard (see page 150) to serve	450 ml	¾ pt	

Grease the inside of a 900 ml/1½ pt/3¾ cup pudding bowl/deep ovenproof bowl thoroughly with a little extra margarine. Put the blackberries into the bowl and sprinkle with 30 g/1 oz of the fructose. Crush the fruit slightly with a fork to free the juices.

In a large mixing bowl, put the margarine and remaining fructose, and whisk until smooth and pale. Add the milk and yogurt mixture, the sifted flour, baking powder, vanilla extract and lemon zest. Beat until thoroughly combined. The batter will be stiff and smooth. In a separate bowl, whisk the egg whites to soft peaks. Fold into the batter, starting with a spoonful to soften the mixture before carefully folding in the rest. Pour the mixture into the pudding bowl on top of the blackberries. Take a length of aluminium foil and fold 4 pleats 2.5 cm/1 in deep along the centre. This will enable the pudding to rise and expand while steaming. Secure with an elastic band. Place the bowl in the top half of a double boiler and steam for 1 hour exactly. Top up the bottom half of the boiler with more hot water from time to time so that it does not boil dry. Meanwhile, make the custard (see page 150).

Remove the pudding from the steamer. Remove the foil. The pudding should be coming away from the sides slightly. Ease a flexible spatula round the edge carefully, so as not to cut into the sponge. Put a serving plate on top of the bowl and carefully invert. Give the pudding bowl a bit of a shake and a tap and the pudding should fall free. Serve immediately with the warm custard.

SERVES 8

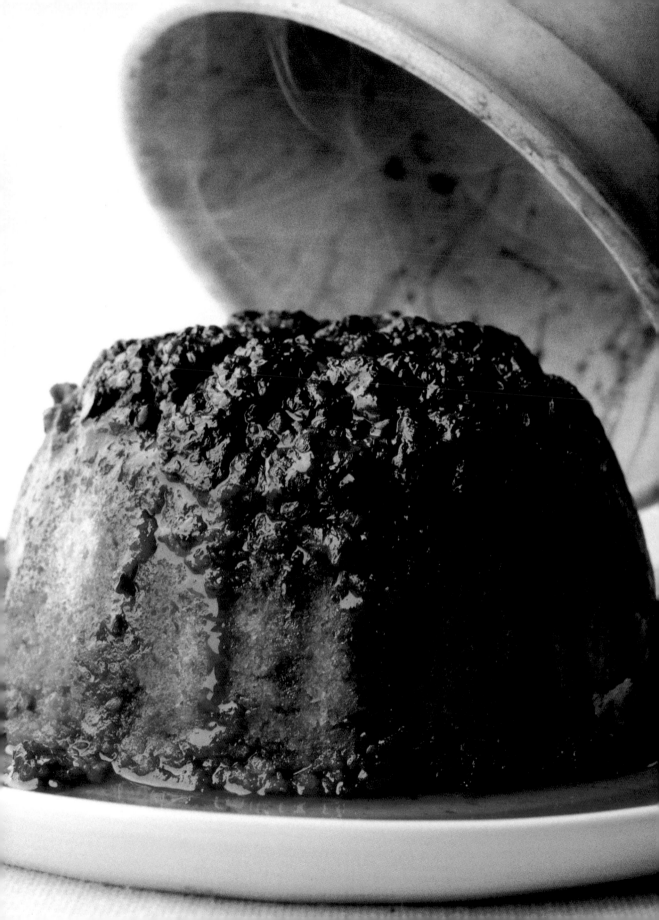

FLAPJACKS

These delicious, easy flapjacks are made using the muesli on page 150. I often bake a batch on Sunday afternoon to take to work on Monday.

	METRIC	IMPERIAL	CUPS
hard margarine	90 g	3 oz	⅓ cup
agave syrup		4 tbsp	
vanilla extract		2 tsp	
muesli (see page 150)	200 g	7 oz	2 cups

Line an 18 cm/7 in square baking tin with greaseproof paper or baking parchment. Preheat the oven to 180°C/350°F/Gas 4.

In a saucepan heat the margarine, agave syrup and vanilla extract until boiling. Add the muesli and stir over the heat for a few minutes. Spoon the mixture into the tin and press down well with a spatula. Bake for 15 minutes.

Remove flapjack from the oven, press down again and return it to the oven for another 5 minutes.

Place on a wire rack to cool and, while still warm, cut into squares. Press down again to firm if necessary and leave to cool completely in the tin. Remove the flapjacks from the tin by lifting the paper. Gently break into squares down the cut lines and store in an airtight container.

MAKES 9 SQUARES

LEMON ICE

I have always shied away from making ice cream, believing that one either needed an ice-cream maker or endless patience, hand stirring the mixture for hours to prevent crystals forming. This recipe requires neither, you simply mix and freeze. The result is a delicious refreshing ice. I would advise freezing the mixture in individual containers to make serving simple.

	METRIC	IMPERIAL	CUPS
juice of 1 1/2 lemons	60 ml	2 fl oz	1/4 cup
sheep's yogurt	500g	1 lb 2 oz	2 1/4 cups
fructose	250 g	8 oz	1 1/4 cups
zest of 1 1/2 lemons (use lemons with unwaxed skins)			

Put the lemon juice in a saucepan and boil. Cool over ice. Bring the yogurt, fructose and lemon zest to the boil, stirring constantly with a balloon whisk, and boil for a minute or two. Remove from the heat. Pour the yogurt mixture into the cold juice. Strain and divide the mixture into individual 'bombe' moulds. Freeze. (Alternatively, the lemon zest may be left in the mixture. It will sink to the bottom and thus appear on the top of the inverted bombes when served.)

Remove the ices from the freezer a few minutes before serving and turn out on to individual plates. Delicious with berries of your choice and the almond cookies on page 118.

SERVES 4

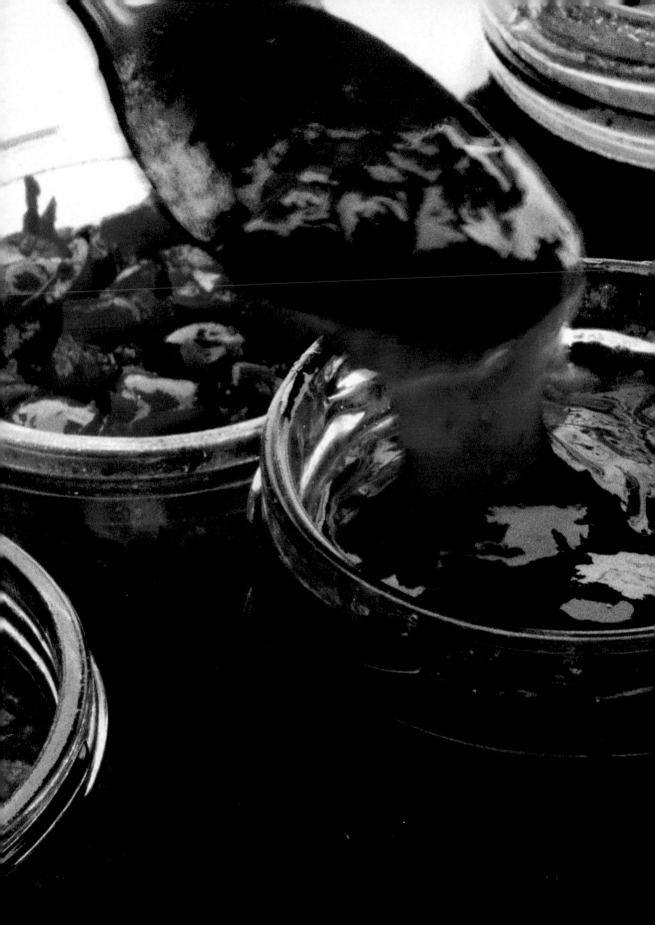

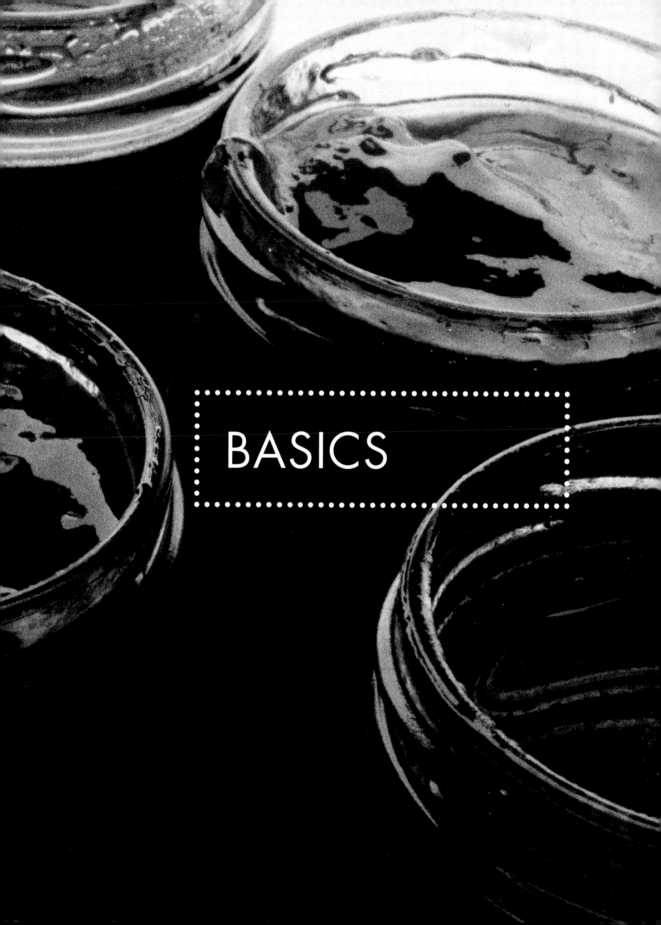

BASICS

DAMSON JAM

One of Terence Stamp's earliest memories was of his mother making damson jam. The wonderful smells of the cooking fruit permeated the house and it was this that really got him first interested in cooking and preparing food.

	METRIC	IMPERIAL	CUPS
damsons	900 g	2 lb	
fructose	350 g	12 oz	1 3/4 cups
water	300 ml	1/2 pt	1 1/4 cups
agar agar (optional)		1/2 tsp	

Wash the fruit and cut through the skins until you reach the stones/pits, as if you were cutting them in half. It is not possible to remove the stones at this point without losing some of the fruit surrounding them. Leave the stones in; they add to the flavour of the jam and will be easy to remove at a later stage.

Put the prepared fruit into a saucepan and sprinkle over the fructose, stirring it in. Set aside for 15 minutes.

Then pour the water over the fruit and bring slowly to the boil. As the stones separate from the fruit, remove them with a slotted spoon. Bring the mixture to a rapid 'rolling' boil and test for the desired set.

If a firm set is required, remove some of the jam juice into a cup and let it cool. Mix in the agar agar, stirring. Bring the jam mixture back to a rapid rolling boil and add the agar agar, stirring briskly. Repeat this process if more set is necessary.

Cool and pour into clean glass jars. Seal and store in a cool place.

BRAMBLE JELLY

This jelly is very quick and simple to make and the degree of set is entirely up to you. It seems that soft set jam is rising in popularity and if this is desired, simply boil the fruit-fructose mixture for less time. Whatever the set, your jam cannot fail to taste delicious. The quantities given are enough to make a small jar of jelly. If you want to make a larger amount, simply multiply the ingredients in proportion.

	METRIC	IMPERIAL	CUPS
ripe blackberries	400 g	14 oz	
apple syrup	60 ml	2 fl oz	¼ cup
water	60 ml	2 fl oz	¼ cup
lemon juice		1 tbsp	
fructose	150 g	5½ oz	¾ cup

Bring the fruit, apple syrup and water to the boil and simmer gently for 30 minutes, crushing the berries from time to time with a wooden spoon. Strain the mixture into a clean pan through a fine plastic or stainless-steel sieve, mashing the fruit with the back of a wooden spoon. Stir in the fructose. Return the mixture to the heat and boil rapidly for about 5 minutes. Test for set.

This is quite a tangy jelly. For a sweeter taste increase the fructose content.

STRAWBERRY JAM

UK legislation states that in order to name a product 'jam' there must be a quantity of sucrose present. Strictly speaking this recipe, and the one for Damson Jam, should be called 'compôtes' because they contain only pure fruit and fructose. As with the Damson Jelly, the quantities here are enough for one small jar – simply multiply them if you wish to make a larger amount.

	METRIC	IMPERIAL	CUPS
strawberries	250 g	8 $\frac{1}{2}$ oz	
fructose	150 g	5 oz	$\frac{3}{4}$ cup
lemon juice		1 tsp	

Hull the strawberries and cut in half, or quarters if the berries are large. Put the fruit into a heavy saucepan over a gentle heat and stir with a wooden spoon until the fruit softens and starts to break up. Remove from the heat when the mixture is half fruit and half purée. Away from the heat add the fructose and lemon juice and stir until the fructose has completely dissolved. Return to the heat, bring the mixture slowly to the boil and then simmer gently for 20 minutes. It will now have reduced and be at the point of setting.

Pour into a clean jar or jam dish. Cool.

CRANBERRY, ORANGE AND CORIANDER SEED RELISH

This is a delicious and pretty standby to serve with pâtés, cold meats and cheeses. Stored in a glass screw-top jar, it will keep for 2 weeks in the refrigerator.

	METRIC	IMPERIAL	CUPS
fresh cranberries	250 g	8 ½ oz	2 ¼ cups
coriander seeds		½ tbsp	
sultanas/golden raisins		1 tbsp	
sunflower oil		1 tbsp	
apple syrup	60 ml	2 fl oz	¼ cup
zest and juice of 1 orange			
ground allspice		¼ tsp	

Crush the coriander seeds in a small bowl with the back of a teaspoon. Do not use the ready ground coriander as it does not have the same 'citrus' qualities.

Put the cranberries, sultanas, oil, syrup and orange juice into a food processor and pulse a few times to chop roughly. Do not overdo this. Alternatively, chop the cranberries and sultanas roughly by hand, placing the chopping board in a tray or baking tin to catch the cranberries because they tend to roll around all over the place!

Put this cranberry mixture into a saucepan with the orange zest, crushed coriander and allspice. Bring to the boil and allow to boil for 2–3 minutes or until the berries soften but are not mushy. Stir and put immediately into a cold dish to help stop the cooking process.

8–10 SERVINGS

CREME A LA VANILLE (CUSTARD)

'Custard' is such an unappealing name and brings back memories of the cold, lumpy, yellow stuff that we had at school. This recipe is properly called *crème à la vanille* and is an altogether different proposition – a pale yellow sauce the consistency of thick cream. This version is adapted from the recipe that I was taught at cooking school. I do not think it can be improved upon, nor is there a simpler method. Purists may wish to exclude the cornflour, however it does help to prevent curdling.

	METRIC	IMPERIAL	CUPS
4 egg yolks			
cornflour/cornstarch		1 tsp	
goat's or sheep's milk	600 ml	1 pt	2 ½ cups
vanilla extract or a vanilla pod/bean		2 tsp	
fructose		2 tbsp	

Put the egg yolks and cornflour into a bowl large enough to hold the milk as well. Set aside.

In a heavy-bottomed saucepan, heat the milk with the vanilla extract or the vanilla pod to the point of boiling. Remove from the heat, remove the vanilla pod if used and whisk in the fructose with a balloon whisk. Cool a little. Break up the yolks with the whisk and pour the slightly cooled milk mixture over the egg yolks, whisking all the time. If the milk is too hot the eggs will scramble.

Return the mixture to the heavy-bottomed saucepan and over a low heat, and stirring constantly with a wooden spoon, heat the mixture until it thickens. Do not allow the mixture to boil. As soon as it is the thickness of cream remove from the heat.

This custard can be served either hot or cold. It will thicken when cold.

SERVES 10

TOASTED MUESLI

I love this for breakfast or as a topping for fruit deserts. The Swiss soak their muesli overnight in fruit juice, which has the advantage of swelling the oats and making them more digestible, but the lovely crunchiness of this version is lost. One of my favourite breakfasts is homemade apple sauce covered with sheep's yoghurt and then sprinkled over with a good helping of this muesli.

In this recipe, the oats are lightly sprayed with apple juice, agave syrup and sunflower oil. The sort of spray used for houseplants is ideal for this. Indeed it is worth keeping one for kitchen use – it's surprising how useful it is.

	METRIC	IMPERIAL	CUPS
jumbo oats or porridge oats	500 g	1 lb 2 oz	6 cups
sunflower oil	100 ml	3½ fl oz	½ cup
apple juice	100 ml	3½ fl oz	½ cup
agave syrup	100 ml	3½ fl oz	½ cup
sesame seeds (optional)	100 g	3½ oz	⅔ cup
sultanas/golden raisins	200 g	7 oz	generous 1 cup

Preheat the oven to 200°C/400°F/Gas 6.

Spread enough of the oats on a baking sheet to form a thin layer. Pour the oil, apple juice and agave syrup into a bottle with spray attachment and shake well to mix thoroughly. Spray over the oats; the more saturated the oats become, the crisper they will end up and can form 'clusters'. (For the calorie-conscious just spray them lightly.)

The cooking time will depend on the amount of coating used but the oats should be lightly golden after about 7 minutes. If the layer of oats is too thick the cereal underneath will not colour and you may need to turn them over, spray again and return the baking sheet to the oven.

Place the toasted oats on a plate to cool and repeat the above until all the oats are toasted.

To toast the sesame seeds (if using), heat a non-stick frying pan/skillet and dry-fry the seeds very lightly indeed, until they only just start to change colour.

Once the oats and seeds are completely cold, put them into an airtight container and mix in the sultanas.

CREME PATISSIERE

This is the basic filling for cold fruit tarts and eclairs. It can be flavoured in different ways with orange zest, cocoa or with almond extract for the French Plum Tart (see page 136).

	METRIC	IMPERIAL	CUPS
3 egg yolks			
fructose	75 g	2 1/2 oz	1/3 cup
cornflour / cornstarch	55 g	2 oz	1/2 cup
goat's or sheep's milk	600 ml	1 pt	2 1/2 cups
2 egg whites			
vanilla extract (or other flavouring)		1 tsp	

In a heavy-bottomed saucepan, whisk the egg yolks, fructose, cornflour and milk together. Cook over a low heat, whisking constantly. As soon as the mixture begins to thicken, remove from the heat and continue to stir. Set aside.

Whisk the egg whites to soft peaks and fold into the custard mixture with the vanilla extract or chosen flavouring.

Return to a gentle heat and whisk constantly until the mixture has thickened and the cornflour has cooked.

Do not be alarmed if the mixture separates. If this happens, strain the crème immediately through a fine sieve into a cold mixing bowl, pressing the mixture through the sieve with a wooden spoon, and whisk vigorously. The mixture will become smooth again.

Chill until required.

BECHAMEL SAUCE

This is the classic white sauce that acts as a base for sauces, soups, soufflés and choux paste, depending upon the amount of flour used. This dairy-free and wheat-free version tastes completely authentic.

	METRIC	IMPERIAL	CUPS
margarine	90 g	3 oz	6 tbsp
Dijon mustard		1 tsp	
all-purpose wheat-free flour		6 tbsp	
goat's milk	500 ml	16 fl oz	2 cups
ground nutmeg			
black pepper			

Melt the margarine in a heavy-bottomed saucepan over a gentle heat. Remove from the heat. Stir in the mustard and flour and blend thoroughly. Using a balloon whisk, stir in the milk and return to the heat, whisking until the sauce reaches the boil and thickens. Continue to boil gently for 3 minutes, stirring constantly to ensure the flour is cooked. Season to taste.

This will give you a smooth, glossy sauce that is thick enough to coat the back of a spoon. For a thinner sauce, add more milk; for a thicker one, less.

For a cheese sauce, add grated cheese to taste off the heat after the sauce has been prepared as above, stirring in vigorously.

VEGETABLE STOCK

This vegetarian stock can be used instead of chicken stock. Almost any vegetables can be used. The skins of the onions should be left on because they give the stock a rich golden colour.

	METRIC	IMPERIAL	CUPS
1 onion			
1 leek			
2 carrots			
2 parsnips			
2 large celery stalks			
2 tbsp olive oil			
boiling water	1.7 litres	3 pt	7 ½ cups
3 sprigs fresh thyme			
3 sprigs fresh parsley			
4 black peppercorns			
3 bay leaves			

Cut the onion into quarters, leaving the skin on. Cut the leek to within 2.5 cm/1 in of the base, open the leaves out and rinse away any dirt under running water. Scrub the rest of the vegetables and cut into chunks, unpeeled if organic, peeled otherwise, with the tops removed.

Put the oil into a large pan adding all the chopped vegetables. Stir to coat with the oil and then cook over a low heat, covered for 10 minutes, stirring once or twice. Pour in the boiling water. Add the herbs, peppercorns and bay leaves, cover and boil gently for 1 hour.

Strain and store in the refrigerator.

CHICKEN STOCK

There are two methods for making chicken stock.

METHOD 1

If a very flavourful, opaque stock is required, follow the previous recipe for vegetable stock, adding the bones, carcass and giblets from a roasted bird when the boiling water is added. Cook, strain and refrigerate as before.

METHOD 2

For a clear broth, do not use any vegetables with the exception of brown onion skin. Put the bones, carcass and giblets into a pan, cover with cold water, bring slowly to the boil and simmer, covered, for 1 hour. The carcass should have completely fallen apart at this stage; if it has not, continue to cook, covered, for another 20 minutes. Strain into a bowl and refrigerate. If a layer of fat forms on the surface of the chilled stock, remove this before using for any recipes that will be served cold.

BASIC SHORTCRUST PASTRY

It is important that the pastry dough be smooth and soft. Adjust the amount of liquid to achieve this texture otherwise the pastry will be difficult to roll out.

	METRIC	IMPERIAL	CUPS
hard vegetable margarine	90 g	3 oz	8 tbsp
all-purpose wheat-free flour	170 g	6 oz	1¾ cups
iced water			

Blend the margarine and flour to resemble crumbs, then bind with enough water to form a ball. Knead the dough for a couple of minutes. If any cracks appear, add more water until the dough is smooth and soft. The water will continue to be absorbed by the flour while the pastry is 'resting' in the refrigerator so err on the side of adding a little extra water. Wrap and chill in the refrigerator for at least 30 minutes.

This can also be done in a food processor. Blend the margarine and flour until the mixture resembles crumbs. Add enough water so that the dough forms a ball. The pastry dough should be soft and smooth with no sign of cracks. Wrap and chill as above.

ACKNOWLEDGMENTS

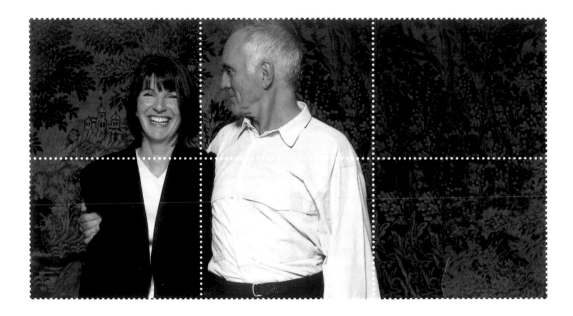

The authors wish to thank the following for their contributions:

Maude Morton
Mark, Poppy and Lucy Buxton
Geraldine West
Jonathan Lovekin
Catherine Calland
Nato Welton
Terry O'Neill
Anthony Michael
Stephanie Nash
Sandra Curtis
Anne Uribe
Greg Lewis
Simon Thomas
Mohamed El Banna
Stephanie Cabot
Charles Levison
Fiona MacIntyre and
Denise Bates

WHEAT-FREE FLOUR

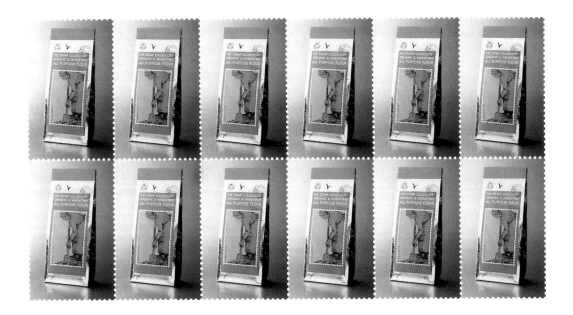

The flour used in these recipes is the Stamp Collection® All Purpose Flour which is 100% organic and 100% wheat-free. When we first talked to our publisher, Fiona MacIntyre, about compiling this cookbook, our recipes included a number of different wheat-free flours: oats, rye, rice, gram, buckwheat, soya, potato, maize and millet, all of which we had become accustomed to using over many years. Fiona pointed out that it would be far easier for cooks to be able to use an all-purpose wheat-free flour. We had also received hundreds of requests from our customers for a wheat-free flour, so we set about developing our own organic blend. This is a carefully balanced mixture of barley, rice, millet and maize. As these recipes show, the flour works equally well in soufflés, cookies, cakes, pancakes and pastries. Cooks will note that the flour absorbs liquids more slowly than regular wheat flour. We would recommend that mixtures are allowed to stand for a few minutes to let the liquids be fully absorbed.

For stockists and mail order information please contact:

Buxton Foods Limited
12 Harley Street
London W1G 9PG

Telephone: +44 (0) 20 7637 5505
Facsimile: +44 (0) 20 7436 0979

e.mail: customerservices@stamp-collection.co.uk
http:/ www.stamp-collection.co.uk

INDEX

Alfalfa Seeds, sprouted, 63
Almonds
Almond Cookies, 118
French Plum Tart with Almond Pastry, 136
Apples
Chicory, Apple, Tomato and Roquefort Salad, 43
Apricots
Roast Quail with Wild Rice, Pine Kernels and Apricot Cakes, 112
Asparagus
Broad Beans, Peas, Asparagus and Spring Onions with Mint, 40
Aubergines
Aubergines and Red Onion with Two Goat's Cheeses, 67
Roast Aubergine, Sweet Potato, Chick-peas and Red Peppers with Spinach, 30
Avocado
Corn, Tomato, Red Onion and Avocado Salad 44

Bananas
Banana and Rhubarb Crumble, 138
Banana and Cinnamon Loaf, 139
Basic Shortcrust Pastry, 155
Beans
Black Bean and Fennel Salad, 46
Duck with Sun-dried Tomatoes and Cannellini Beans, 115
Spicy Bean Soup, 18
Steamed Tofu and Spiced Sprouted Beans, 64
see also Broad beans; Green beans
Béchamel Sauce, 153
Black Bean and Fennel Salad, 46
Blackberries
Bramble Jelly, 147
Steamed Blackberry Pudding, 140
Blinis, 26
Braised Red Cabbage, 32
Bramble Jelly, 147
Broad Beans, Peas, Asparagus and Spring Onions with Mint, 40
Buckwheat Kasha Salad with Halloumi Cheese, 52

Cabbage, Braised Red, 32
Cake
Carrot, Pineapple and Walnut Cake, 132–4
Chocolate Cake with Roasted

Hazelnuts, 128
High Tea Fruit Cake, 127
Caper Berries
Skate with Caper Berries and Black Olives, 84
Carrots
Carrot, Pineapple and Walnut Cake, 132–4
Sweet Potato and Carrot Soup, 17
Celeriac and Leek Frittata, 60
Char-Grilled Tuna Steaks with Mint Salsa Sauce, 80
Cheese
Aubergines and Red Onion with Two Goat's Cheeses, 67
Buckwheat Kasha Salad with Halloumi Cheese, 52
Cheese and Garlic Soufflé, 58
Cheese Triangles, 122
Chicory, Apple, Tomato and Roquefort Salad, 43
Potato Gratin, 39
Swiss Chard Gratin, 29
Chicken
Chicken Niçoise, 94
Chicken Stock, 155
Creamed Chicken with Coconut and Aromatic Spices, 98
Green Chicken, 110
Lemon Tarragon Chicken with Button Mushrooms, 100
Marinated Roast Chicken Breasts, 99
Quick and Easy Chicken Liver Paté, 24
Roast Chicken, 95
Roast Chicken with Okra Provençal, 96
Chick-peas
Roast Aubergine, Sweet Potato, Chick-peas and Red Peppers with Spinach, 30
Tuna and Chick-pea Salad, 90
Chicory, Apple, Tomato and Roquefort Salad, 43
Chilli
Vegetarian Chilli, 50
Chocolate Cake with Roasted Hazelnuts, 128
Clam Chowder, 12–13
Coconut
Creamed Chicken with Coconut and Aromatic Spices, 98
Crème à la Vanille (Custard), 150
Cod with Jalapeño Pepper and

Dill Coating, 91
Cookies
Almond Cookies, 118
Fresh Ginger and Honey Cookies with Pine Kernels, 120
Corn
Corn, Tomato, Red Onion and Avocado Salad, 44
Corn Chowder, 20
Crispy Corn Fritters, 28
Crab
Crab Cakes, 86
Cranberry, Orange and Coriander Seed Relish, 149
Creamed Chicken with Coconut and Aromatic Spices, 98
Crème Patissière, 152
Crispy Corn Fritters, 28
Crumble, Banana and Rhubarb, 138
Curry, Mixed Vegetable, 34
Custard
Crème à la Vanille, 150

Damson Jam, 146
Date and Walnut Muffins with Orange Zest and Nutmeg, 124
Double-Crusted Nectarine Pie, 130
Duck
Duck Terrine with Green Peppercorns, 22
Duck with Sun-dried Tomatoes and Cannellini Beans, 115
Wild Duck with Fennel, 114

Eggs
Red Camargue Rice and Roast Vegetables with Eggs, 54–5

Fennel
Black Beans and Fennel Salad, 46
Mussel, Parsnip, Fennel and Leek Ragout, 76
Wild Duck Braised with Fennel, 114
Fish, 73–91
Fish Pie, 82
Flapjacks, 142
Flour, Wheat-Free, 157
Fowl, 93–115
French Plum Tart with Almond Pastry, 136
Fresh Ginger and Honey Cookies with Pine Kernels, 120

Fritters
Crispy Corn Fritters, 28
Grated Potato, Pea and Spring
Onion Fritters, 62
Fruit Clafoutis, 135

Garlic
Cheese and Garlic Soufflé, 58
Parsnip and Garlic Mash, 42
Scallops with Garlic Potatoes,
Watercress and Red Onion, 88
Ginger
Fresh Ginger and Honey Cookies
with Pine Kernels, 120
Puy Lentils with Ginger, 25
Roast Turkey Thigh with Honey and
Ginger Glaze, 102
see also Japanese ginger
Gougère, 106–7
**Grated Potato, Pea and Spring
Onion Fritters**, 62
Green Beans
Green Beans with Cherry Tomatoes,
33
Green Chicken, 110
Green Salad, 47
Guinea Fowl and Turnip, 111

Hazelnuts
Chocolate Cake with Roasted
Hazelnuts, 128
High Tea Fruit Cake, 127
Honey
Fresh Ginger and Honey Cookies
with Pine Kernels, 120
Roast Turkey Thigh with Honey and
Ginger Glaze, 102
Sesame Seed and Cherry Honey
Squares, 119

Ice, Lemon, 143
Individual Mushroom Soufflés,
38

Jam
Bramble Jelly, 147
Damson Jam, 146
Strawberry Jam, 148
Japanese ginger
Roasted Salmon with Sultanas and
Japanese Ginger, 74
Salmon Tartare with Japanese
Ginger, 36

Leeks
Celeriac and Leek Frittata, 60
Mussel, Parsnip, Fennel and Leek
Ragout, 76
Lemon
Lemon Ice, 143
Lemon Tarragon Chicken with Button

Mushrooms, 100
Lentils
Lentil Soup, 16
Puy Lentils with Ginger, 25
Liver
Quick and Easy Chicken Liver Paté,
24
Liz's Lunch Tortilla, 66

**Maple Syrup and Sultana
Scones**, 131
**Marinated Roast Chicken
Breasts**, 99
Mint
Broad Beans, Peas, Asparagus and
Spring Onions with Mint, 40
Char-grilled Tuna Steaks with Mint
Salsa Sauce, 80
Pea and Mint Soup, 14
Mixed Vegetable Curry, 34
**Monkfish and Stuffed
Mushrooms**, 78–9
Muesli
Toasted Muesli, 150
Muffins
Date and Walnut Muffins with
Orange Zest and Nutmeg, 124
Mushrooms
Individual Mushroom Soufflés, 38
Lemon Tarragon Chicken with Button
Mushrooms, 100
Monkfish and Stuffed Mushrooms,
78–9
Mushroom and Morel Soup, 35
Wild Mushrooms and Autumn
Vegetables with Potato Cakes,
68–70
**Mussel, Parsnip, Fennel and
Leek Ragout**, 76

Nectarine Pie, Double-Crusted,
130

**Oatcakes with Sesame Seeds,
Scottish**, 123
Okra
Roast Chicken with Okra Provençal,
96
Olives
Skate with Caper Berries and Black
Olives, 84
Onions
Aubergines and Red Onion with
Two Goat's Cheeses, 67
Corn, Tomato, Red Onion and
Avocado Salad, 44
Scallops with Garlic Potatoes,
Watercress and Red Onion, 88
Three Onion Risotto, 56
see also Spring Onions
Orange

Cranberry, Orange and Coriander
Seed Relish, 149
Date and Walnut Muffins with
Orange Zest and Nutmeg, 124
Watercress and Orange Salad, 43

Parsnips
Mussel, Parsnip, Fennel and Leek
Ragout, 76
Parsnip and Garlic Mash, 42
Pastry
Basic Shortcrust Pastry, 155
French Plum Tart with Almond Pastry,
136
Pasta
Penne Gratin, 51
Seafood Spaghetti, 87
Paté
Quick and Easy Chicken Liver Paté,
24
Peas
Broad Beans, Peas, Asparagus and
Spring Onions with Mint, 40
Grated Potato, Pea and Spring
Onion Fritters, 62
Pea and Mint Soup, 14
Penne Gratin, 51
Peppers
Roast Aubergine, Sweet Potato,
Chick-peas and Red Peppers with
Spinach, 30
Pheasant Braised with Plums,
108
Pine Kernels
Fresh Ginger and Honey Cookies
with Pine Kernels, 120
Roast Quails with Wild Rice, Pine
Kernels and Apricot Cakes, 112
Plums
French Plum Tart with Almond Pastry,
136
Pheasant Braised with Plums, 108
Potatoes
Grated Potato, Pea and Spring
Onion Fritters, 62
Potato Bake, 71
Potato Gratin, 39
Scallops with Garlic Potatoes,
Watercress and Red Onion, 88
Squid and Potato Stew, 75
Wild Mushrooms and Autumn
Vegetables with Potato Cakes,
68–70
Puddings
Steamed Blackberry Pudding, 140
Pulses, sprouted, 63
Puy Lentils with Ginger, 25

Quails
Roast Quails with Wild Rice, Pine
Kernels and Apricot Cakes, 112

Red Cabbage, Braised, 32
Red Camargue Rice and Roast Vegetables with Eggs, 54–5
Relish
Cranberry, Orange and Coriander Seed Relish, 149
Rhubarb
Banana and Rhubarb Crumble, 138
Rice
Red Camargue Rice and Roast Vegetables with Eggs, 54–5
Roast Quails with Wild Rice, Pine Kernels and Apricot Cakes, 112
see also Risotto
Risotto
Three Onion Risotto, 56
Roast Aubergine, Sweet Potato, Chick-peas and Red Peppers with Spinach, 30
Roast Chicken, 95
Roast Chicken with Okra Provençal, 96
Roast Quails with Wild Rice, Pine Kernels and Apricot Cakes, 112
Roast Turkey Thigh with Honey and Ginger Glaze, 102
Roasted Plum Tomatoes, 42
Roasted Salmon with Sultanas and Japanese Ginger, 74

Salad
Black Bean and Fennel Salad, 46
Buckwheat Kasha Salad with Halloumi Cheese, 52
Chicory, Apple, Tomato and Roquefort Salad, 43
Corn, Tomato, Red Onion and Avocado Salad, 44
Green Salad, 47
Tuna and Chick-pea Salad, 90
Watercress and Orange Salad, 43
Salmon
Roasted Salmon with Sultanas and Japanese Ginger, 74
Salmon Tartare with Japanese Ginger, 36
Sauce, Béchamel, 153
Scallops with Garlic Potatoes, Watercress and Red Onion, 88
Scones
Maple Syrup and Sultana Scones, 131
Scotch Pancakes, 126
Scottish Oatcakes with Sesame Seeds, 123
Seafood Spaghetti, 87
Sesame Seed and Cherry

Honey Squares, 119
'Shepherd's Pie', 104
Skate with Caper Berries and Black Olives, 84
Soufflés
Cheese and Garlic Soufflé, 58
Individual Mushroom Soufflés, 38
Soup
Clam Chowder, 12–13
Corn Chowder, 20
Lentil Soup, 16
Mushroom and Morel Soup, 35
Pea and Mint Soup, 14
Spicy Bean Soup, 18
Sweet Potato and Carrot Soup, 17
Spaghetti
Seafood Spaghetti, 87
Spicy Bean Soup, 18
Spicy Seafood Stir-fry, 83
Spinach
Roast Aubergine, Sweet Potato, Chick-peas and Red Peppers with Spinach, 30
Spinach Tart, 59
Spring Onions
Broad Beans, Peas, Asparagus and Spring Onions with Mint, 40
Grated Potato, Pea and Spring Onion Fritters, 62
Sprouted Pulses and Seeds, 63
Squid and Potato Stew, 75
Steamed Blackberry Pudding, 140
Steamed Tofu and Spiced Sprouted Beans, 64
Stew, Squid and Potato, 75
Stock
Chicken Stock, 155
Vegetable Stock, 154
Strawberry Jam, 148
Sweet Potatoes
Roast Aubergine, Sweet Potato, Chick-peas and Red Peppers with Spinach, 30
Sweet Potato and Carrot Soup, 17
Swiss Chard Gratin, 29

Taramasalata, 21
Tarragon
Lemon Tarragon Chicken with Button Mushrooms, 100
Tarts
French Plum Tart with Almond Pastry, 136
Spinach Tart, 59
Terrine
Duck Terrine with Green Peppercorns, 22
Three Onion Risotto, 56
Toasted Muesli, 150
Tofu

Steamed Tofu and Spiced Sprouted Beans, 64
Tomatoes
Chicory, Apple, Tomato and Roquefort Salad, 43
Corn, Tomato, Red Onion and Avocado Salad, 44
Duck with Sun-dried Tomatoes and Cannellini Beans, 115
Green Beans with Cherry Tomatoes, 33
Roasted Plum Tomatoes, 42
Turkey Burgers with Spicy Tomato Sauce, 103
Tortilla
Liz's Lunch Tortilla, 66
Tuna
Char-grilled Tuna Steaks with Mint Salsa Sauce, 80
Tuna and Chick-pea Salad, 90
Turkey
Roast Turkey Thigh with Honey and Ginger Glaze, 102
'Shepherd's Pie', 104
Turkey Burgers with Spicy Tomato Sauce, 103

Vegetables
Mixed Vegetable Curry, 34
Vegetable Stock, 154
Red Camargue Rice and Roast Vegetables with Eggs, 54–5
Wild Mushrooms and Autumn Vegetables with Potato Cakes, 68–70
see also names of vegetables
Vegetarian main dishes, 49–72
Vegetarian Chilli, 50

Walnuts
Carrot, Pineapple and Walnut Cake, 132–4
Date and Walnut Muffins with Orange Zest and Nutmeg, 124
Watercress
Scallops with Garlic Potatoes, Watercress and Red Onion, 88
Watercress and Orange Salad, 43
Wheat-free flour, 157
Wild Duck Braised with Fennel, 114
Wild Mushrooms and Autumn Vegetables with Potato Cakes, 68–70